Return to Wholeness

Embracing Body, Mind, and
Spirit in the Face of Cancer

David Simon, M.D.

John Wiley & Sons, Inc.

New York • Chichester • Weinheim • Brisbane • Singapore • Toronto

The information contained in this book is not intended to serve as a replacement for professional medical advice. Any use of the information in this book is at the reader's discretion. The author and the publisher specifically disclaim any and all liability arising directly or indirectly from the use or application of any information contained in this book. A health care professional should be consulted regarding your specific situation.

Library of Congress Cataloging-in-Publication Data:

Simon, David
    Return to wholeness : embracing body, mind, and spirit in the face
of cancer / David Simon.
        p. cm.
    Includes bibliographical references and index.
    ISBN 0-471-29577-9 (hardcover : alk. paper)
    1. Cancer—Alternative treatment. 2. Medicine, Ayurvedic.
I. Title.
RC271.A62S54 1999
616.99'406--dc21   98-18402

Printed in the United States of America
10 9 8 7 6 5 4 3 2 1

To my beloved children,

Max and Sara.

May wholeness be your companion all the days of your lives.

In memory of

Jill Simon Bernstein,

whose presence and absence

changed our lives forever

Contents

9 A Time to Every Purpose, 142
Harmonizing with the Rhythms of Nature

10 Emotional Healing, 153
Riding the Turbulent Wave of Feelings

11 Healing through Expression, 173
Deepening Insight through Drawing and Movement

Foreword
by Deepak Chopra

Life is a magnificent paradox. We are ultimately spiritual beings vibrating as conscious energy while appearing as physical entities made of flesh and blood. When we primarily identify ourselves with our physical bodies, localized in time and space, subject to the laws of entropy and decay, we are susceptible to fear, anguish, and disease. When we remember our true nature as Spirit, the veil of ego-based ignorance is parted and we glimpse our essential Self as eternal, boundless, and whole. Whether you think of yourself as physically fit or are in the midst of a life-threatening illness, the most valuable gift any loved one or healer can provide you is the reminder that the *real* you cannot succumb to illness and cannot die.

In this beautiful book, *Return to Wholeness*, written by my dear friend and colleague Dr. David Simon, readers are inspired and encouraged to awaken their inner healer, which is the basis of all personal transformation. With love, compassion, and sensitivity, David reminds us that facing our mortality offers a window into our immortality. A reservoir of energy, creativity, and vitality resides within us all, and the very practical tools offered in this book enable us to tap into its healing waters.

The approaches in this book have been demonstrated to have powerful life-affirming effects at the Chopra Center for Well Being in La Jolla, California. Dr. Simon has helped guide many hundreds of people with cancer along their healing journey in our *Return to Wholeness* program, which is now being offered in health care institutions around the country. It is my fervent hope and belief that this book will help catalyze a genuine transformation in our approach to illness that integrates the best of Western medical technology along with a reverence for and understanding of our profound natural healing forces. If you are facing cancer or any other serious illness, I encourage you to allow the wisdom contained within these pages to nurture, guide and support you. I am grateful that David has written a book that so clearly helps shepherd us back to our source—our birthright of wholeness.

Acknowledgments

Many loving souls have participated in the birth of this book, including family members, close friends, colleagues, and patients. To each of you who have graciously shared your joys and sorrows, strengths and vulner-abilities, insights and feedback, with me, I offer my deep appreciation.

I wish to express special gratitude to:

Stephen Bickel, Danielle Dorman, Jeremy Geffen, and Gayle Rose,

Deepak and Rita Chopra,

Muriell Nellis and Jane Roberts,

Tom Miller,

Myron, Lee Shirley, Howard, Dana, Samantha, Melissa, Judy, Al, Bruce, and Lori,

And my darling wife, Pam, whose loving reflection makes me whole.

Introduction

In the clarity of a quiet mind, there is room for all that is actually happening and whatever else might also be possible.—RAM DASS

You learn you have cancer, and in that moment, your life changes. A torrent of feelings is unleashed into consciousness. Disbelief, dismay, anguish, and dread grapple for dominance in your awareness—one distressing emotion transforming into another without clear boundaries. Each of these feelings is the mask of a more primordial emotion: *fear.* Fear of pain, fear of disfigurement, fear of dependency, fear of regret, fear of loss, fear of death. And with the activation of this most basic emotion, a chemical cascade of stress hormones—the result of millions of years of evolution—floods your body, inciting you to fight or run.

Unfortunately, unlike a furtive stranger in a dimly lit alley, the provocateur of your panic is not outside of yourself, and there is no place to escape this threat. Rather, you feel betrayed by your own cells, and this disloyalty adds another level of anguish and despair. Core questions arise in your agitated mind: How could this be happening to me? What did I do to deserve this? What's going to happen to me? Who will take care of my children? Am I going to die?

These reactions to learning you have cancer are natural. Although we intellectually accept that our physical bodies will eventually break down, it is invariably a shock when we learn we are facing a serious illness. It is a rare person who is able to casually navigate the turbulent sea into which cancer casts us. And yet, in the midst of this unwanted storm lies an opportunity for deep insight into life. I hope to inspire and encourage you with the thought that through the power inherent in your heart and mind, you can steer a course to a place of profound healing.

Almost immediately upon learning of your condition, you must engage in the process of delineating your illness and plotting a therapeutic strategy to address it. With this, a new series of questions often arises: What more can I do to improve my outcome? How can I stimulate my inner healing response to maximize the benefit of my medical treatments?

1

How can I be an active partner rather than a passive participant in my therapeutic journey?

This book, *Return to Wholeness*, is written for those who are asking these questions. It is dedicated to educating and empowering people facing cancer so they can improve the quality, and quite possibly the quantity, of their lives. It is not a book promoting alternative approaches for cancer as a substitute for the best of Western medical care, for I deeply believe that appropriately utilized medications, surgery, and radiation treatments are as much a part of holistic cancer care as good nutrition, herbal medicines, and guided imagery. However, it is clear that many people facing cancer have physical, emotional, and spiritual needs that are not being addressed in modern oncology programs. *Return to Wholeness* seeks to help fulfill these needs.

~

Discovering that you or a loved one has cancer is a life-transforming event. Cancer automatically and instantaneously thrusts you and your loved ones into a time of crisis. In Chinese, the word for crisis, *Wei-ji*, is a fusion of the symbols for danger and opportunity. Although no one consciously chooses to develop a serious illness, many people look back and see their challenge with cancer as the most important and meaningful experience of their lives. In view of the many distressing feelings coursing through you since hearing your diagnosis, the suggestion that this illness may at some point be seen as a gift may seem unimaginable. Yet, with a new perspective, this unintended journey may yield opportunities for personal growth and wisdom that nourish your body, mind, and spirit in unprecedented ways.

My goal in this book is to guide you along the unfamiliar terrain you will encounter in your therapeutic journey. By providing you with the understanding and tools to access your powerful reservoir of inner healing, I hope to offer you genuine encouragement that you can positively influence the course and meaning of your illness. Your thoughts, emotions, and life choices are capable of creating an inner and outer healing environment.

I am not suggesting that if you simply assume a mood of cheerfulness or repeat affirmations your cancer will magically evaporate. Rather, what is required is a genuine shift in perception that creates the opportunity for a new interpretation of the challenge facing you. An understanding of the mind-body connection supports the idea that our perceptions and interpretations of the world around us—the sounds, sensations, sights, tastes, and smells—are translated into the chemical codes that orchestrate our body's symphony of energy and information. Whatever we allow into our mind-body network—be it chemotherapy, nutritious food, balancing herbs, soothing music, or loving emotions—transforms the very substance of our life and can mean the difference between well-being and suffering, between life and death.

Our interpretation of every event in our lives ultimately becomes our record of reality, and our expectations for the future are influenced by our memories and interpretations of the past. If we have watched friends or family members struggle with cancer, our expectations will be shaped by that experience. Yet, it is important to remember that there are as many different responses to cancer as there are people confronting this illness, and many have successfully navigated their way back to health.

The ability to learn new ways to perceive and interpret life's challenges is the great gift of being human. We can move beyond reflexive and reactionary modes of response and use our creativity to give birth to new solutions. If we are willing to make changes in our approach to life, we can incorporate new ways to enliven our healing response. The force of evolution embraces the possibility for solutions that have not been previously tried. Throughout this book I emphasize that our choices can make a real difference. We can be active participants in our recovery. We can learn to consciously invoke the wisdom of Nature—the ultimate source of all healing.

~

My interest in healing goes back a long way. Before I entered medical school, I studied anthropology in college, focusing on how healing was supported in societies around the world. I learned that in almost every culture on earth, illness was viewed as a loss of integration between body, mind, and spirit. Recovery of health required looking for the point of disruption in this continuum and reactivating the connection. The loving support of family and community, mythic reenactments to evoke emotional insight, and spiritual rituals to connect the patient with a higher power were as essential as medicines, nutritional support, and physical therapies. The doctor's expertise was not only in understanding the disease but also in guiding his patients in discovering the psychological and spiritual meaning of their illness.

When I entered medical school, I was disappointed to discover that this broader concept of illness and health was barely acknowledged in Western scientific medicine. Searching for ways to integrate the emotional and spiritual aspects of medicine, I investigated a vast array of alternative

medical systems. Acupuncture, the Alexander technique, applied kinesiol-
ogy, aromatherapy, Bach flower remedies, chiropractic, craniosacral therapy, herbal medicine, homeopathy, macrobiotics, Qi Gong, Reiki, Rolfing,
sacro-occipital technique, Shiatsu, therapeutic touch, Traeger, and more—
in each I discovered an acknowledgment of a vital life force that tran-
scended material reductionism; still, I felt a need for a unifying framework
that embraced all healing modalities.

When I discovered Ayurveda, the traditional medical system of India,
I felt I had reached the Promised Land. Ayurveda, which means "life science," offers a holistic framework for healing that embraces body, mind,
and spirit. It is not the specific Himalayan herbs or massage techniques
that distinguish Ayurveda from other systems; rather, it is the all-
encompassing perspective that enables us to integrate healing modalities
ranging from psychic surgery to neurosurgery. A classic story about Jivaka, the Buddha's personal physician, illustrates the holistic nature of
Ayurveda. While applying for a faculty position at an Ayurvedic medical
college, Jivaka was given the assignment to find substances that could
not be used medicinally. Several days later, he returned empty-handed,
saying he could not find a single substance that had no potential therapeutic value. Every flower, tree, and weed, every mineral and creature,
the wind, sun, and sea—all had potential healing properties when used
appropriately.

"When the only tool in your toolbox is a hammer, everything looks
like a nail" is an expression that can easily be applied to health care today.
Medical doctors use medicines, acupuncturists use needles, chiropractors
use adjustments, and each works in a certain situation. The value that
Ayurveda brings is not so much as another alternative modality, but
rather that it is a common language into which every healing discipline
can be translated. Ayurveda sees life as the exchange of energy and information between individuals and their environment. If our environment
provides nourishment, we thrive; if our environment offers toxicity, we
languish. Therefore, learning how to transform toxicity into sustenance
is the key to health and healing.

Throughout this book I will be using Ayurvedic concepts but have
chosen mainly to avoid Sanskrit terminology, with the intent of eliminating any barriers to gaining the most benefit from these holistic principles. For those interested in diving deeper into this expansive body of
knowledge, an Ayurvedic suggested reading list is provided in the Ap-
pendix. I deeply believe the ageless wisdom traditions can add tremendous value in our search for greater well-being, and I hope this book

demonstrates the limitless benefits of integrating the ancient and modern healing traditions.

~

Although trained as a neurologist and not an oncologist, I have personally supported hundreds of patients facing cancer. Whether primarily directing the treatment of people with tumors of the nervous system or developing mind-body programs for people facing cancer at the Chopra Center for Well Being, I have repeatedly been impressed by the spiritual opportunity that serious illness affords. Cancer impels us to confront our mortality and, in so doing, to embrace our immortality. When we encounter the real possibility of death, our entire conception of time is altered. Unresolved issues from the past and material goals for the future lose much of their importance. Each day takes on new meaning and purpose as our priorities realign from material to emotional to spiritual issues. Those aspects of our life that have limited or transitory value fade in importance, while those core to our meaning rise to the forefront.

I commonly see estranged families reuniting when a member has cancer. I often see people who have recovered from cancer leave jobs they've been dissatisfied with for years and pursue dreams they've carried their whole lives. And, with rare exceptions, people facing serious illness strive to discover the deeper meaning of their lives, consciously stepping onto a spiritual path that offers the hope of eternity.

In *Return to Wholeness*, I hope to convince you of something very radical. You—the real you—do not have cancer. Your body may have malignant cells, your mind may be defining you as a "cancer patient" or "cancer survivor," but the essential nature of who you are is beyond illness. You are not a physical machine with the ability to generate consciousness, feelings, and ideas. You are a localized field of intelligence in a vast universe of consciousness. You are consciousness made manifest. . . . At your core, you are Spirit, and as such you cannot become sick and you cannot die.

A sacred song from the Upanishads declares:

In the city of Brahman is a secret dwelling, the lotus of the heart. Within this dwelling is a space, and within that space is the fulfillment of our desires. What is within that space should be longed for and realized. . . .

Never fear that old age will invade that city; never fear that this inner treasure of all reality will wither and decay. This knows no age when the body ages; this knows no dying when the body dies. This is the real city of Brahman; this is the Self, free from old age, from death and grief, hunger and thirst.[1]

Diane Connelly once said, "All sickness is home sickness." The simple truth of this statement suggests that healing is the process of coming home. Where is home? It is not our body and it is not our mind, for these aspects of ourselves are in constant and dynamic flux. Home is the source of all our thoughts and feelings, it is the basis of our being, it is the field of awareness that unites us with all existence. Our essential nature is wholeness and holiness. I hope that this book will help you rediscover your home, pointing the way so that you may return to wholeness.

CHAPTER 1

Understanding Cancer

Through the Windows of Modern Science and
the Timeless Healing Traditions

The merging of intuition and reason will provide wisdom for the resolution of the struggle in which we are engaged.—JONAS SALK

As a young child, I used to imagine a bogeyman living under my bed. I was certain that this beastly troll waited to materialize until my parents turned off my bedroom lamp. I envisioned him hungrily anticipating my placing one foot onto the floor, eager to devour my tender, though meager, body. If I needed to empty my bladder after I had been officially tucked into bed, I would go to elaborate extremes to avoid touching the floor, climbing over dresser tops and bounding across cushioned chairs to the doorway. I could not even consider the idea of looking under the bed to see if there was really something there to stoke my fears. On some level I enjoyed the danger and the challenge of outwitting my fearsome goblin.

It would be wonderful to believe that cancer could be avoided if we were only clever enough to sidestep its underhanded ways. Although cancer is in many ways the bogeyman of our society, this disease cannot be evaded by illusion or delusion. Cancer challenges us at every level of life—environmentally, physically, emotionally, intellectually, and spiritually. If we are to understand and move beyond cancer, we must be willing to look into its face and resolutely commit to hearing its message.

Cancer is a disease of our age. Every time I release exhaust fumes from my car, purchase a tomato that does not have a trace of insect damage, or fail to recycle a plastic container, I contribute to our collective risk for cancer. It has been estimated that over 80 percent of cancers are environmentally influenced.[1] This includes not only obvious environmental factors such as tobacco, asbestos, and ultraviolet radiation but also takes into account the risks of the high-fat diet that is the staple of most Americans. And it is almost impossible to account for the harmful effects that modern stress has on our immune system's ability to recognize and eliminate malignant cells.

Cancer is a complex process, which involves some factors that we can control and others that we cannot. Like the prayer for Alcoholics Anonymous, it's helpful to know which things we can change, which things we can't, and how to tell the difference. The foods we eat, the toxins we knowingly ingest, the ways we use our five senses, and how we express our emotions—all are under our control. We can choose to accept only life-affirming influences and eliminate toxic ones.

Our genetic constitution, which includes our inherited vulnerability to illness, is beyond our conscious control. Similarly, the air we breathe, the water we drink, the chemicals in our soil, the toxins in our workplace, and the electrical fields that surround us are for the most part not within our personal control but represent our collective tolerance for toxicity in our environment. Awareness of our intimate relationship with the ecology of our earth is reawakening, and soon we will have a critical mass of people committed to improving the quality of life on our planet. As this unfolds, our standards for personal and environmental purity will be transformed, and cancer will be understood in a new light.

Discovering Cancer

My brilliant friend, Dr. Candace Pert, one of the pioneers in the field of mind-body medicine, uses an amusing slide in her medical presentations. It features the tombstone of a person who lived for ninety-five years, with the inscription "You see, it wasn't psychosomatic!" I see many people each year whose fear of cancer erodes their day-to-day quality of life. A woman who watched her mother's battle with breast cancer believes it is only a matter of time before she suffers a similar fate. A man whose older brother had colon cancer becomes obsessed with his bowel function, certain that every episode of constipation portends a malignancy. People who have a heightened fear of cancer seem to take one of two routes. In one, they torment themselves about every bodily symptom, certain that it is heralding a serious problem. They frequent their physician's office, convinced that this time they will receive the bad news they have been anticipating.

The other approach is to deny the problem, hoping that by ignoring a symptom it will disappear. A woman with fibrocystic breast disease feels a small swelling but refuses to bring it to the attention of her doctor. She worries about it constantly but avoids dealing with it directly. Much more often than not, the mammogram she finally agrees to is completely normal, and she realizes she has expended months of needless anguish.

The anxiety associated with this illness can be as devastating as the illness itself. I recently saw a woman at the Chopra Center who was convinced that she had thyroid cancer. She tearfully told me that ten years earlier her family doctor had noticed a slight swelling in her neck. Although he had *not* raised the possibility of cancer, she became convinced that this was her problem and avoided any medical care from that point on, terrified that her fear would be confirmed. When I examined her, I could not find any problem. When I asked her how long ago she had last felt the lump, she stated that it had been almost ten years ago! Despite the complete absence of any physical abnormality, this woman had lived her last decade in misery, afraid that her life was going to be shortened by cancer.

Throughout this book I will be advocating a middle path. As we enter the twenty-first century, denying the value of modern medical advances is as regrettable as denying the healing value of herbs. Although this book is dedicated to using holistic approaches to help people who are directly facing cancer, I fully support the use of the early detection technologies we have available. Regular physical examinations, mammography, prostate specific antigen (PSA) levels, cervical Pap smears, skin examinations, and rectal examinations with tests for occult blood are important tools for detecting cancers at earlier and more treatable stages. If you notice a change in your body, pay attention! Denial and delay do not ultimately serve the healing process. If something is awry, find out what it is and what therapeutic options are available to you. Most important, find a health care advisor you can trust to guide you compassionately and expertly through the thicket of choices available. Despite how scary it may feel to face our challenges directly, it is ultimately the only path to true healing.

Looking at Cancer from a Consciousness-based Mind-Body Approach

Later in this chapter, I'll explain the current scientific understanding of what cancer is, how it develops, and what is usually done in modern medicine to combat it. First, I'd like to look at cancer in a different way. This new approach seeks to understand the message cancer is bringing to us as individuals and society. This perspective generates a series of questions that we need to explore openly if we are to move beyond the suffering that cancer brings.

What is the deeper meaning of this illness that creates so much anguish?
What is cancer telling us about the way we are living our lives?
What can we do to change the impact cancer is having on us, as individuals and as a community?

These are big questions without easy answers. However, searching for the meaning of cancer is a worthy quest that offers potential treasures that may be unimaginable to you at this time. My hope is that throughout this book, the questions raised will motivate you to look deeply into your own mind, heart, and soul to discover the meaning of the challenge cancer brings.

Let's first explore what's happening when the body functions in a healthy manner. It's really a miracle that the trillions of cells in our body, all derived from a primordial fertilized egg, are able to carry out their millions of life-sustaining functions in a coordinated fashion. Each cell has a very specific role, while simultaneously contributing to the wholeness of the mind-body physiology. Our liver cells are capable of detoxifying our blood, storing and releasing sugar molecules, and metabolizing cholesterol while at the same time monitoring the levels of dozens of hormones, digesting hemoglobin pigment, and reproducing daughter cells. Just a short distance away, our colon cells are absorbing fluid, propelling the residue of yesterday's lunch along, and monitoring the concentration of bacteria. Throughout the body, our cells, the fundamental building blocks of life, are performing their myriad tasks in a coordinated manner that is beyond our conception of organizational power.

In every timeless healing wisdom tradition is the recognition of a life force that unifies and coordinates biological intelligence. In Traditional Chinese Medicine it is referred to as *chi* and is described as life energy that circulates through subtle channels known as meridians. This is the basis of acupuncture treatments designed to remove obstacles to the free flow of this vital force. In Ayurveda, the primary energy that creates and sustains life is known as *prana*, meaning "the primary impulse." As long as prana is flowing, life is maintained. When the body is no longer capable of functioning in the coherent way that supports the flow of life force, the individual life ends. A body immediately before and after death is composed of the same set of biochemicals, but life contains the unifying vital force that animates our molecules into a living, breathing being.

What is this unifying force that organizes a complex set of biochemicals into a human being with awareness and the ability to think, feel, and act? This question is at the heart of the new paradigm of life and health that is blossoming in our society as we undergo the transition from a material to an information- or consciousness-based perspective. After two hundred years of a worldview that considered only physical reality to be worthy of attention, the dawn of the information age is heralding a new vision that embraces consciousness as a real force. As these new principles permeate society, a new approach to health and illness is emerging.

On my first day of medical school almost twenty-five years ago, I began my study of health by dissecting a human cadaver. The implicit message that my colleagues and I received was that the key to understanding health begins with the understanding of death and illness. I say implicit because in most modern medical schools there is only limited discussion of the basic philosophy of life and death, health and disease. Rather, most institutions make the assumption that future doctors of medicine understand their role to be master technicians of disease. According to the prevailing model taught in medical colleges, life is the product of complex chemical reactions that generate awareness, ideas, and emotions as by-products of molecular reactions. Death is then viewed as the inevitable end of a faulty biological machine (the human body), similar to the breaking down of an old automobile.

The problem with this material approach to life is not so much that it is wrong, but that it is incomplete. The most brilliant scientists of our time tell us that the world is not as solid as it may seem. Through the insights of the great physicists of the twentieth century, we now understand that underlying the facade of matter is a very mysterious nonmaterial world. Although to our senses the environment appears as a collection of individual solid objects, we now know that the atomic building blocks that comprise this domain of forms are mostly emptiness. The relative distance between an electron and the nuclear core of an atom is as vast as the distance between stars in our galaxy. Even the subatomic particles that make up atoms are ultimately nonmaterial, for as soon as we try to precisely locate them in space, they vanish into a cloud of probability. According to the timeless tradition of Ayurvedic science, the entire universe of forms and phenomena is a temporary consolidation of a nonmaterial field of energy and information. All this matter is ultimately nonmatter.

The Ayurvedic message and the message of modern physics are remarkably resonant with one another. Albert Einstein cognized the formula $E = mc^2$, convincing the world that matter and energy are interchangeable. As scientists continue delving into the quantum soup that underlies the world of perception, we are learning that an invisible potential reality gives rise to the building blocks that structure our universe. The womb of creation is beyond the limits of time and space, but its nature is to give birth to time and space. Physicists have referred to this nonmaterial field of potential energy and information that gives rise to the world as the unified field, or the vacuum state. Ayurvedic scientists call it the field of pure potentiality, the field of pure consciousness, or in Sanskrit, *Brahman*. We can also call it the field of infinite possibilities, because all that was, is, or will be arises from this field.

A consciousness-based approach takes another step here, suggesting that the same field of intelligence that underlies the world around us is the basis of our own awareness. The steady stream of thoughts and feelings that we experience consists of impulses of intelligence emerging from a nonlocal field of awareness. The field of pure potentiality that gives rise to subatomic particles, rainbows, and galaxies gives rise to our creativity, ideas, and emotions. Rather than consciousness being the by-product of molecules colliding in our brain, our thoughts and cells are both expressions of this underlying field of intelligence. Our physical body is a field of molecules; our mind is a field of ideas, but underlying both our mind and body is a field of consciousness that gives rise to both. In the timeless wisdom traditions, this field of consciousness is also referred to as spirit.

Our life force is the expression of the infinite organizing power of spirit that provides the unifying coherence to the cells of our body. Our connection to the universal field of intelligence enables each of our cells to express its unique properties while simultaneously supporting the wholeness of our physiology. However, when there is some interference in the free expression of the intelligent vital force within us, the coherence between our cells becomes disrupted. The memory of wholeness is forgotten, and individual cells begin acting as if they are disconnected from the body as a whole. According to a consciousness-based model, this is the origin of cancer. Due to the accumulation of toxic influences or cellular misunderstandings, an individual cell assumes a level of self-importance that disregards its cellular community. The cancer cell reproduces, failing to recognize that in its uncontrolled expression of power it is sowing the seeds of its own destruction.

Searching for Meaning

Let's revisit the first question raised earlier, "What is the deeper significance of this illness that creates so much anguish?" I suggest that all persons who are affected by cancer—whether as patient, family member, friend, or health care provider—ask this question in their own minds and listen to the answers from their hearts. At the Chopra Center, the procedure we have found most helpful is to have people close their eyes, allowing their attention to go inward to their heart. Then the question is quietly asked and each person silently listens to the response that emerges from within his or her own awareness. Ideally, try this exercise with someone who is going through your journey with you. Sit quietly with your eyes closed, centering your awareness in the region of your heart. After a minute of silence, have your partner softly whisper in your ear, "What is the deeper significance of this illness?" every fifteen or twenty seconds. Listen without preconception to the information that emerges. The more innocent you can be in listening to, rather than forcing, a response, the more your inner wisdom will emerge. After hearing the question and listening to your inner message several times, take a few minutes to write down what you learned.

Your first thought may be that there is no deeper significance to this terrible disease and that you simply want it to vanish from your life as rapidly as possible. This is fully understandable, for no one consciously chooses to incur an illness. However, most people who perform this exercise receive some insights that begin the process of regaining meaning and wholeness in life. Often, people with cancer, as is true with most people on this planet, can identify some aspect of their life that is incomplete in some way. That is, they know that there is something missing but have been unable or unwilling to address this lack directly and may necessary choices to improve the situation. It may be that you are languishing in a job that provides little nourishment or challenge. It may be that you are harboring resentment or bitterness from a past or current relationship. It may be that you have a desire to spend more time with your family members but other priorities always seem to win out. Perhaps a change in diet or a new exercise program has been calling you, but you have done everything in your power to tune out the message. It may simply be some hobby such as painting, writing, or dance that always brings you great joy, yet you never seem to have time for it. Almost all of us would make different choices if we really believed that our time here was limited. For many people, learning that they have a serious illness offers the opportunity to look honestly at what is missing and to begin choosing to fulfill that need.

About one and a half years ago, a frightened woman with breast cancer came to see me, understandably distraught because her cancer had recurred nine months after a malignant breast mass had been surgically removed. After her operation, her surgeon told her that her chances for a cure were excellent, and she declined further treatment. Unfortunately, a lump that was at first felt to be scar tissue from the surgery continued enlarging, and a repeat biopsy showed more malignant cells. After her first round with cancer, she did her best to put the experience behind her as quickly as possible, treating the whole episode as a bothersome inconvenience. She continued to smoke cigarettes, made no changes in her fastfood diet, and remained in a less than nourishing relationship with her boyfriend, even though he was unable to provide emotional support for her when her illness was discovered. When she discovered that the cancer had returned, her emotional defenses were overwhelmed, and she was terrified that she was going to die. She was prepared to do anything that might improve her chances. Working with her oncologist, she began a program of radiation, chemotherapy, and hormonal therapy, along with several mind-body approaches. She learned meditation, improved her diet, and gave up smoking. When she asked herself what was the deeper significance of her illness, her quiet inner voice told her that her cancer represented a lack of love for herself. Recognizing a long-standing pattern of one-sided relationships, she made a commitment to herself that she would no longer tolerate emotional toxicity in her life. A year and a half later, she is disease-free, in a healthy relationship with a wonderful man she met at a cancer support group, and happier than she has been in many years. In retrospect, she sees her cancer as a gift that impelled her to make choices honoring her spirit.

I will be reminding you throughout this book to give yourself permission to nurture your innermost desires and live your life as if every moment was a gift. We each have a responsibility for our own well-being, and in order to create health, we need to restore the wholeness that is our birthright. Responsibility is not the same as blame. We often hear from people with cancer that well-meaning friends attempt to convince them they are choosing to create their illness, implying that if they simply chose differently, they could spontaneously eliminate their illness. This is neither useful, compassionate, nor accurate. Regardless of the specific choices we make in our lives, one thing is certain—no one chooses to suffer. Even people who smoke two packs of cigarettes a day are not choosing to get sick; rather, they are choosing a behavior that fulfills a need they have not found another way to satisfy. People are often willing to dispense with life-damaging habits when life-supporting alternatives are offered.

Whenever my patients raise the issue of what they did to cause their cancer, I feel a tremendous amount of humility and compassion. First, they may not have done anything on a conscious level to incur their illness. Children of Hiroshima who developed leukemia, adults with thyroid cancer who were radiated for swollen tonsils as children, and women with vaginal cancer exposed in their mother's womb to the hormone diethylstilbestrol (DES) can hardly be held personally accountable for their cancers. These reflect our collective choices more than any one individual's. Second, there are many types of cancer for which we do not understand how any of our conscious behaviors contribute to their development. Although there may be statistical correlations between certain types of environmental influences and specific cancers, for many malignancies we simply don't have the "why" answers. This is certainly the case for the many people I see with brain tumors. Third and finally, there is no value in creating any sense of blame in people who are now facing the most important challenge of their lives. I suspect that by assigning a simplistic cause to an effect ("Of course he got colon cancer, he ate red meat!") we protect ourselves from the fear that serious illness raises in us. If my friend who works too hard gets sick, I can feel some security that since I do not indulge in that behavior, I am protected from a similar fate. In my experience, humility and compassion are the qualities that truly benefit friends when someone is facing cancer or any other serious life challenge.

More important than assigning blame is assuming the responsibility to create an opportunity for healing. By responsibility I mean the *ability* to *respond* in a creative way that is different from the past and open to new possibilities. Only through escaping the limitations of the past can we access our full creative potential. This means looking at every aspect of our lives and honestly evaluating whether we are maximizing nourishment or tolerating toxicity. Through honest self-evaluation we gain the power to make the changes that will bring about greater happiness and well-being in our lives. This is true whether or not we are currently facing a serious illness. Acknowledging our limitations or weaknesses does not mean that we are flawed; rather, the recognition that we are multifaceted human beings allows us to embrace the paradoxical aspects of our nature. Cancer can be viewed as a dramatic wake-up call to us as individuals and society. In our reawakening, we can restore wholeness to our lives.

What Is Cancer?

Since I will be using medical terminology throughout this book, I'd like to familiarize you with a few basic definitions. Recognizing that the language we use to describe something determines our relationship to it, I will be introducing new ways of describing cancer that will help shift our interpretation of cancer. But I think it is useful to understand the prevailing terminology of this illness.

Let's consider a common scenario. You become concerned about a swelling under your arm and see your doctor about it. He examines the lump and labels it a *tumor*, which simply means a swollen collection of cells. The question in both your and your doctor's minds is whether the tumor is *benign* (most likely harmless) or *malignant* (potentially serious). If your doctor is unable to confidently determine the nature of the swelling by feeling it, he will probably recommend a *biopsy*—an operation to take all or a piece of the tumor so it can be examined under a microscope.

You obviously hope the lump is benign. Benign tumors are usually slow-growing, don't spread throughout the body, and are unlikely to shorten life. They have well-defined boundaries, separating them from surrounding healthy tissue. When an operation is performed to remove a benign tumor, none of the cells in the lump are usually left behind.

You fear that the tumor is malignant. This implies that it is more rapidly growing, has a tendency to invade healthy tissue, can spread, or *metastasize*, and may be threatening to life. Because malignant tumors do not heed the normal boundary rules of the body, it may be more difficult to determine where the lump ends and normal tissue begins.

If the biopsy shows only an increased number of normal cells, the lump is declared benign and no further treatment is required. If, however, the microscopic examination shows cells that seem to be multiplying beyond normal controls, the scary diagnosis of *cancer* is applied. The term *cancer* is derived from the Greek word *karkinos*, meaning crab, because malignant tumors tend to hold onto surrounding tissues like a stubborn crab.

If the tumor is malignant, you will probably be referred to a doctor who specializes in the treatment of people with cancer, known as an *oncologist*. Most modern treatment offered by an oncologist falls under one of three categories: surgery, chemotherapy, or radiation therapy. The goal of a surgical procedure is to remove as much of the cancerous tissue as possible, minimizing the damaging effect it has on surrounding normal tissue. Chemotherapy involves the use of potent medicines that damage cells that are rapidly growing. Since cancerous cells tend to reproduce more quickly than normal healthy cells, chemotherapy drugs are designed to affect malignant tissues more than normal ones. Because there is not an absolute distinction between the way normal and cancerous cells grow, it is normal for people receiving chemotherapy to experience some side effects. Radiation therapy involves directing beams of energy at cancerous tumors, which alter their genetic material, leading to cell death. As with chemotherapy, the goal with radiation treatments is to maximize the effect on cancer cells while minimizing injury to normal cells. Two modalities that hold promise for the future are immune therapies that enhance our body's ability to identify and dispense with cancer cells and genetic treatments that seek to correct the abnormal signals that stimulate cancer cells to grow. The newest approach on the horizon uses substances known as angiogenesis inhibitors that may treat cancer by preventing the development of new blood vessels. If a tumor cannot augment its blood supply, it cannot grow. Preliminary research in animals using these agents is promising, and the cancer community eagerly awaits studies in human beings.

Many cancers are effectively treated with modern medical approaches, but because medical doctors are reluctant to use the term *cure*, people who have a good response to treatment are usually referred to as going into *remission*. In complete remission, all evidence of cancer is gone; in partial remission, the cancerous tissue may be lessened but still detectable at some level. A tumor that seems to have stopped growing or is growing much more slowly than expected may also be considered to be in partial remission. By reducing the burden of cancer cells with modern medical treatment, your body's natural healing system has a better chance of taking care of the remaining malignant cells.

Environmental Agents

Over the past several decades scientists have tried to understand how toxic substances can lead to cancer when they enter our bodies. The term *carcinogen* is applied to an agent from the environment that may stimulate the uncontrolled growth of cancer cells. For most carcinogens, a minimum exposure is necessary before a person develops cancer. For example, many soldiers fighting in Vietnam were exposed to Agent Orange, a poison used to destroy forests. Limited exposure to the chemicals contained in Agent Orange, known as dioxins, rarely led to cancer, but workers heavily exposed to the herbicide where it was produced have shown a higher risk for a number of malignancies. Even with the same carcinogen exposure, human beings demonstrate a wide range of susceptibility to developing cancer, based upon both our genetic makeup and our overall state of health. We can't do much about our heredity, but we can do a lot to improve our overall health.

Cancer, Lifestyle, and Culture

As a life insurance actuary, Thomas knew that his pack-per-day cigarette habit was placing him at some health risk, and each year he made a resolution to stop. However, his day-to-day life stresses always provided a good reason why today was not the right day to begin enduring the anticipated nicotine withdrawal symptoms. Although annoyed by his chronic cough, he avoided seeing his doctor until one morning when he was startled to see his urine appearing pink in the toilet bowl. Anxiously describing his discovery to his family doctor on the telephone, he was scheduled to see a urologist that afternoon. After a series of studies, he was given the diagnosis of bladder cancer. Fortunately, it was small, localized, and very treatable.

A year later, Thomas is a changed man. He smoked his last cigarette on that fateful day, lost thirty unwanted pounds, now

exercises four times a week, and regularly enjoys family vacations. He looks back with a sense of gratitude on the experience
that helped him reset his physical and emotional priorities.

Almost any tissue in our body can be the site of cancer, because
everywhere our cells grow there is the potential for them to lose normal
control and reproduce in a disorganized manner. The most common tumors in any given culture or community reflect the prevailing popular
lifestyle. For example, lung cancer is the most common malignancy in the
United States because of our society's addiction to tobacco. If no one
smoked cigarettes, lung cancer would be a rare disease. Unfortunately, as
more women in our society choose to smoke, what was previously a rare
malignancy in women is now common. Equally tragic, the incidence of
tobacco-related cancers is growing worldwide as citizens of developing
countries emulate our Western lifestyle.

Our digestive system is almost continuously exposed to carcinogens
in our environment through the food we consume. Nearly half of all cancers in the United States arise within the digestive tract, with the large intestines the most common site. High dietary fat intake and low fiber
consumption are associated with slower movement through our gut, which
seems to increase the exposure of our colon to potential cancer-causing
substances. Diet has a major effect on this type of cancer, as shown by the
fact that the rate of colon cancer in North Americans and Western Europeans is as much as ten times higher than in natives of Asia, Africa, and
South America![2] In Seventh-Day Adventist communities, where members tend toward vegetarianism, the incidence of colon cancer is much
lower.[3] Native Japanese have a high incidence of stomach cancer, apparently related to the large amount of salted, pickled, and smoked foods
that comprise the typical Japanese diet. Japanese people who move to
Hawaii or California and change their diet to a more characteristically
American one show a decrease in the incidence of stomach cancer but a
rise in their risk of colon cancer.[4]

Our modern lifestyle not only raises the risk of some cancers; it lowers the risk of others. Liver cancer is relatively rare in North America,
where it is usually related to long-standing alcoholism. However, developing countries in Africa and Asia have a very high incidence of liver cancer. Malnutrition, exposure to toxins produced by food contaminated by
fungus, and a variety of viral and parasitic infections may all contribute to
the phenomenal 8 percent incidence of deaths due to liver cancer in
southern Africa.[5] We can fairly easily reduce the risk of liver cancer

through lifestyle choices in North America. The societal changes required in the poorest developing countries are much more challenging.

Breast and prostate cancer are of major concern in North America. Although we do not understand why we are having epidemics of these cancers, they seem to be related to our lifestyle. Both breast and prostate cancer are much less common in Asia. As with colon cancer, when women move from Japan to America, the risk of breast cancer rises, as does the risk of prostate cancer in Asian men who move here.[6] The rising rate of breast cancer in America has been tied to a diet rich in animal fat, and this has also been confirmed in studies on animals. We know that women who never have children or who have their first child after the age of thirty have a slightly higher risk of breast cancer. Women on estrogen replacement therapy are also at mildly increased risk. These trends are more common among Western women, accounting in part for the increased breast cancer we see here. There has also been recent concern about toxic chemicals known as endocrine disruptors. A variety of environmental agents may mimic or alter our natural sex hormones, possibly contributing to breast, prostate, and testicular cancer.[7] The Environmental Protection Agency is sponsoring studies to more carefully assess the role of these common chemicals in our most common cancers.

Although environmental factors have been identified in many cancers, there is still much we don't understand. A thousand people may be working in the same chemical plant, but only a handful will develop cancer. Millions of people smoke packs of cigarettes each day, but not everyone develops lung, mouth, or throat cancer. This is where two other important issues come into play: genes and immunity.

Genes and Cancer

Richard was understandably concerned when during a screening examination, several small polyps were discovered in his colon, as both his father and older brother had died in their sixties of colon cancer. Fortunately, the biopsy report was benign for all the tumors removed. Wanting to do everything possible to avoid the fate that had taken his family members, he learned that he could reduce his cancer risk by making some changes in his diet. He stopped eating red meat and increased the fiber in his diet. Reducing his salt intake, he made certain to have several daily servings of fresh fruits and vegetables, rich in antioxidants and potassium. He also cut back on his alcohol intake. Although he could not change his genetic predisposition, he could improve his chances through regular examinations and simple nutritional changes.

Our DNA molecules contain millions of years of evolutionary information on how to create a living, working cell. Shortly after our father's sperm merges with our mother's egg cell, the genetic blueprints of our parents pair up, creating the biological map of our life. The script that describes the color of our eyes, the texture of our hair, the shade of our skin, and many of our personality characteristics is written in our code of life, waiting to be translated from the interwoven threads of our genes. The instructions for the essential proteins that form the building blocks of our cells and tissues unfold sequentially in a miraculous choreography of feedback loops. Genes affect every aspect of cellular function, including growth, maintenance, repair, and dissolution.

Normal cells follow orderly patterns of growth and development, responding to environmental influences in ways that maintain balance and health. They have well-defined boundaries and produce offspring only when necessary. Cancer cells, however, do not observe the regulations of the body. They do not honor the boundaries designed for harmony and order and instead reproduce without concern for the needs of surrounding cells and tissues.

Studies over the past twenty years have shed light on how the usual cellular control mechanisms can break down in cancer cells as a result of genetic alterations. When the genetic information of a cell is changed as a result of inherited or acquired damage, several possibilities arise. One possible consequence is that the cell is too changed to survive, in which case it systematically self-destructs. Another possibility is that the genetic alteration is so minor that the cell performs less efficiently, but not enough to cause either death or abnormal growth. Most of the time we will never notice these first two changes, since our overall health is not affected. However, if a genetic alteration affects growth-regulating proteins, the cell may stop listening to normal control mechanisms, signaling the onset of cancer.

The genes that are responsible for stimulating cells to reproduce are called *proto-oncogenes*. These are our growth-promoting genes, which are essential at various stages of a cell's life. During our earliest development from a single cell to a complex multidimensional being in the womb, our growth genes provide the driving force to produce the trillions of cells that comprise our bodies. Whenever there is an injury to a tissue, our growth genes are activated, stimulating cells to reproduce and repair the damage. Tissues that are normally rapidly changing, such as our skin and blood-producing cells, are under the constant stimulation of growth-promoting genes.

The problem arises when these growth-promoting genes turn on but fail to turn off. When these blueprints for growth are altered through exposure to a virus or environmental toxin, they may continue to stimulate reproduction even though there is no healthy need for growth. When normal growth-promoting genes are altered so that they continue to stimulate uncontrolled growth, they are called *oncogenes*—genes that cause cancer.

Another important component of the cancer picture is a set of genes that are designed to shut *off* cellular growth. These are called *tumor suppressor genes*, because when they are altered, they become incapable of turning cell growth off. Both oncogenes that stimulate cells to divide and tumor suppressor genes that stop cells from dividing are often involved in cancer. It is now believed that most cancer starts with a single cell that undergoes two or more genetic alterations over many years before it begins growing uncontrollably. This "two-hit hypothesis" explains why it may take years of exposure to a carcinogen such as cigarette smoke before a person develops cancer. Because a cell's DNA must undergo at least two different mutations before it loses control, our body's repair system must be overcome twice in the same gene for cancer to arise. Considering the hundreds of thousands of genes in our cells and the trillions of cells in our body, the odds of this occurring are fortunately fairly low, but the longer we are exposed to a toxic substance, the higher the odds become. This also explains why it is still beneficial to stop after years of smoking, because the likelihood of another cancer-producing mutation in our genes is then reduced.

As was true in Richard's case, certain forms of cancer run in families, suggesting that they carry an inherited susceptibility. One possible explanation for these families is that their inherited weakness is in the genes that repair DNA damage. We are all exposed on a daily basis to cancer-causing influences but we do not all develop cancer. This is because we have an elaborate genetic repair system that scans and repairs defects before the cell is allowed to reproduce. It's as if we have a genetic spell-checker that identifies and corrects any misspelled DNA words before the story is printed. Families with inherited tendencies toward cancer seem to have weak repair systems so that over time, potential cancer-causing misspellings have a higher chance of showing up.

Cancer and Immunity

Our immune system is an elaborate network of cells and messenger molecules designed to identify and eliminate unwanted biological intruders. Although we will explore this area in greater detail in the next chapter, I'd like to present a few basic principles here. Each of our normal cells has identifying proteins that let our immune system know they are friendly. These proteins can be thought of as an identification card. If a foreign organism enters our system, our immune cells immediately ask to see its identification card, and if it cannot produce the right ID, an alarm is triggered, provoking our immune cells to respond. Whenever we inhale or ingest a virus or bacteria, it is identified as familiar or alien by comparing the trespasser's characteristics with those of prior invaders. If the alien is identified as unfriendly, chemical signals are released that mobilize the appropriate immune troops.

Our immune system has a variety of different cells designed to disarm and disable any biological invader that may cause harm to us. Some immune cells release protein antibodies that immobilize the foreigner, others secrete chemicals that disrupt its protective lining, and still other cells engulf the intruder like hungry crocodiles. In each case, the end result is the neutralization of the intruder.

Most of the time, our amazing system of immunity functions beautifully, providing us with a protective brigade from the horde of innumerable environmental challengers that surround us. Similarly, our immune system usually protects us from internal challenges by identifying and eliminating cells that have undergone genetic changes. This component of immunity is known as our *cancer surveillance system*. When a cell undergoes a gene change, it is usually noticed by our immune system and promptly deactivated. Many oncologists believe that each of us creates several potentially malignant cells each day that never develop further because of our cancer surveillance system. However, cancer cells are normal cells that have been transformed, not foreign invaders. Because of this, they may not be as easily identified as potentially harmful by our immune system. In other words, cancer cells' identification cards may be altered, but our immune cells may have to look very closely to see that there is something false about them.

Malignant cells may also develop the ability to hide their distinguishing marks until they have reproduced for several generations. Once cancer cells have taken hold, it becomes more difficult for our immune system to deactivate them. Most people with cancer then require the more powerful treatments of surgery, radiation, and chemotherapy to reduce the burden of cancer cells so the immune system can regain the upper hand.

As we will be discussing throughout this book, one of the aims of mind-body approaches is to support the immune system so that it can be a stronger partner in the treatment of cancer. We now know that the immune system can be weakened or strengthened by our moods, emotions, and states of mind. Changing our perceptions and interpretations of the experience of cancer and its treatment can make a major difference in both quality and quantity of life. Understanding that our internal dialogue can profoundly influence our immune system opens new possibilities for healing.

Commitment to Wholeness

Our bodies are the end product of our experiences and interpretations. To change our bodies, we need to change our experiences. Make a commitment to change your life in the direction of greater love and caring for yourself and those close to you.

1. I consciously choose to eliminate toxic influences and to accept only nourishing influences in my life. I do not blame myself for choices that I made in the past, recognizing that I am doing my best at every moment.

2. I will ask what is the meaning of this illness and listen openly to my quiet inner voice. I will take action to increase the joy in my life.

3. I will consider all therapeutic approaches available and work in partnership with my health care advisor to create an optimal healing program.

CHAPTER 2

Eavesdropping on the Mind-Body Conversation

How Our Mind and Our Body Communicate in Health and Disease

One who knows the self is dear will cherish and protect it; the wise one is vigilant through the night.—BUDDHA, IN THE DHAMMAPADA

Terrence, the immune T cell, was on night shift duty guarding the breathing passages. It had been a pretty uneventful evening. He caught a few rowdy pollen particles attempting to sneak into a bronchial tube, but they were easy to shoo off without much fuss. Things were so quiet that Terrence was starting to drift off when suddenly he was aroused by a coughing sound. Without warning, a gang of strep bacteria surrounded him. Caught off guard, he quickly sounded his alarm, calling for backup help. Within minutes Bertha, the immune B cell, arrived and immediately began releasing her immobilizing antibodies against the invading germs. Norman, the natural killer cell, and Marvin, the macrophage, were on the scene a few moments later. As a team, the immune squad was able to quickly apprehend the thugs before they caused any real trouble. Terrence learned an important lesson that night, vowing never to be caught napping on the job again.

Our immune system has one primary function—to discriminate between self and nonself. Our immune cells vigilantly screen each new visitor to our body, deciding whether it is friend or foe. If an alien virus or bacteria has the capacity to create mischief, our well-tuned immune system promptly incapacitates it. If an immune cell has not previously met the foreigner, it checks its cellular memory bank, looking up the historical account of an ancestral encounter. Our immune sentry cells are continuously weighing whether to sound an alarm or allow the stranger to pass.

Just because something is new does not automatically mean that we need to mount a defensive response. An unfamiliar food may provide valuable nutrition, pollen from an imported flower may offer no threat, and saliva from a lover may nourish us like nectar. Our immune cells may simply note the characteristics of the exotic substance and let it go by without reaction. However, when a foreign agent has a history of causing injury, our biological defenses are mobilized.

For every challenge, there is an ideal response, with the intensity of our reaction proportionate to the offense. If we respond lazily to a threat, we may suffer unnecessarily. Alternatively, if we respond in an overly aggressive way, our reaction may cause more harm than the provocation itself. Balance and appropriateness are the hallmarks of a healthy response to any challenge in life. And this is certainly the case for our immune system. If we underrespond to a virus or bacteria, the resultant infection causes suffering and depletion of our energy. If we respond excessively to an external challenge, we may suffer needlessly, as when we have allergic reactions. There is nothing inherently dangerous about the pollen of an acacia tree, but if my immune cells sound the alarm when its flowers are in bloom, I pay the price with sneezing, scratchy eyes, and a runny nose.

Our immune system is also responsible for continuously monitoring our internal environment, checking the identity cards of cells on our host team. Our normal cells carry on their surfaces proteins that identify their place of origin. Most of the time when these markers are present, our immune cells are not aroused. Occasionally, however, for reasons that we don't understand, apparently normal cells trigger immune reactions, resulting in inflammatory responses against healthy cells. It may be that foreign proteins on viruses or bacteria are close enough to normal ones that our immune cells become confused, unable to distinguish ally from enemy. This is the basis of autoimmune diseases such as rheumatoid arthritis and multiple sclerosis.

On the other end of the spectrum, our immune system may not respond aggressively to signals that herald a possible malignancy. There are two possible explanations for this nonchalant reaction. One is that our immune cells are not sufficiently alert to the subtle changes that cancer cells express. The other possibility is that the cells that have undergone a cancerous alteration are skillful at hiding them from our immune system. Let's explore the immune system a little more deeply to understand how we might help it perform optimally.

The Actors in the Immune Drama

Jonas Salk, the great American physician who developed the first polio vaccine, used to wonder what the world looked like from the perspective of a virus or a cancer cell.[1] This stimulated his creativity, leading to experiments that tested his imagination. In a similar way, I find that personifying the lives of immune cells helps me better understand the immune process.

There are four major characters in the immune drama: T cells, B cells, natural killer cells, and macrophages. Each plays an important role in our defense against outside and inside challenges.

1. T Cells (Terrence). T cells develop in our thymus gland, which overlies our heart. There are two major types of T cells—those that stimulate other immune cells (helper cells) and those that subdue them (suppressor cells). T cells are like platoon sergeants, leading the troops into battle when there is a threat and holding them back when fighting is unnecessary. They communicate primarily through messenger molecules called *cytokines*. There are dozens of these communicator chemicals that can stimulate cells to multiply, incite them to fight, or encourage them to calm down. It's as critical to turn off an immune response when the task has been completed as it is to activate a response when a battle is at hand.

2. B Cells (Bertha). When a B cell learns there is a potentially harmful alien in the system, it quickly becomes excited and begins making antibodies, which are small proteins that attach to other molecules. Once production is in gear, B cells release their antibodies into the circulation like torpedoes or heat-seeking missiles going after a target. We have thousands of different lines of B cells, which can create and release antibodies against a vast array of potential aliens. When one of these antibody

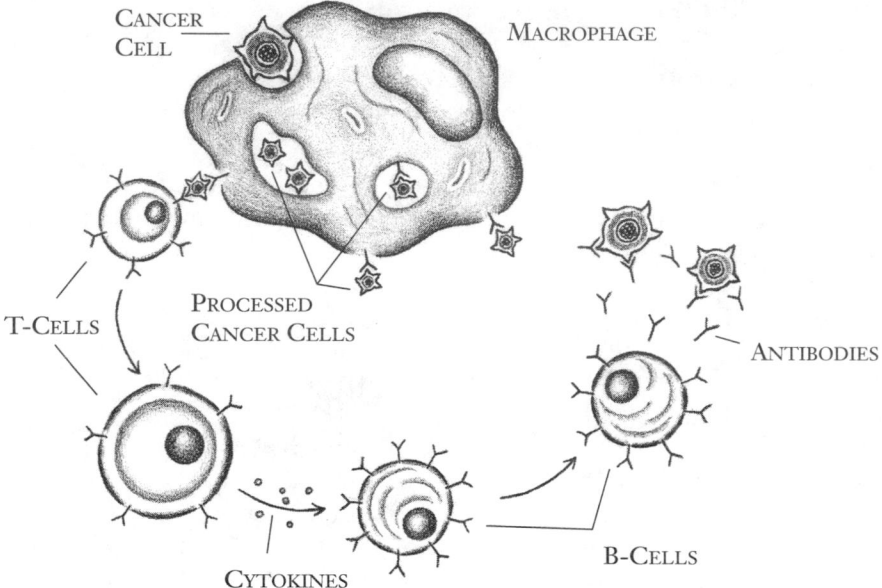

Figure 1 **Immunity and Cancer**

missiles attaches to an invading structure, it makes it easier for other immune cells to identify, disable, and digest the intruder.

3. Natural Killer (NK) Cells (Norman). When natural killer cells are activated, they attach to alien cells, releasing little packets of chemicals that punch holes in and digest the protective covering of the intruder. They bind to the antibody missiles released by B cells and vigorously respond to many of the chemical messengers released by T cells. NK cells play an important role in our immunologic response to cancer.

4. Macrophages (Marvin). The word macrophage means "big mouth," which aptly describes this cell that gobbles up alien invaders. This is the cell that is sometimes visualized as a living Pac-Man, devouring bacteria, viruses, and cancer cells. Like natural killer cells, macrophages are aroused by B cells, whose antibodies make targeted creatures more digestible, and T cells, which send out appetite-enhancing chemicals.

With these four powerful brigades available, how is it possible for tumor cells to escape detection and elimination? We are just beginning to learn how cancer cells evade our immune system. Our immune cells are ambivalent about how aggressive they should be in attacking cancer cells, because they are not entirely foreign. Although most cancer cells express foreign markers, they also express normal ones. It's as if they're double agents with two different passports, and the border guards aren't sure whether they should arrest them or let them pass. There is also a suggestion that cancer cells shed copies of their foreign proteins in the blood, which act like decoys confusing our immune cells. Finally, cancer cells may learn to mimic the chemicals that can sedate an immune reaction, like a burglar feeding hamburger laced with a tranquilizer to a guard dog. With all these possible tricks up the sleeves of cancer cells, we can see how important it is that we function at our optimal level of immunity. Mind-body approaches can enhance our mental and physical well being, sending appropriate support messages to our immune system.

Mind, Body, and Immunity

Ask any grandmother if our states of mind influence our physical health, and she'll probably have stories about Uncle Manny who had a heart attack after his business failed, or Cousin Laura who developed cervical cancer after her husband left her. Although almost all of us have noticed that we are more likely to get sick when we're exhausted or under stress, medical science has been slow to recognize the connection between our mental and physical well being. However, over the last several years there has been an explosion of fascinating information that not only confirms the mind-body connection but also offers interesting explanations for how it works.

This story has actually been slowly unfolding over the past fifty years, since physiologists discovered that when we perceive a threat from our environment, our brains release a cascade of hormones that stimulate our body to respond. Some of these chemical messengers cause our heart to speed up and our blood pressure to rise. Others stimulate our liver to release sugar, providing energy for our tissues. Still other hormones send messages to our immune cells, sounding the alarm for them to respond. These dramatic changes prepare us to react vigorously to a potentially life-threatening challenge in one of two ways: fight or flight. If I'm walking in the jungle and a boa constrictor crosses my path, the alarm I feel in my mind quickly translates into an active response of either grabbing a big stick or hightailing it away from there.

The threats facing us in our modern urban jungle are not so dramatic, but they are equally harmful. The frequent daily stresses of rush hour traffic, time-pressured work deadlines, volatile relationships, and financial pressures take their toll on our emotional well being. The repeated activation of our stress response creates a harmful effect on our immune system over time. Hans Selye, the noted Canadian doctor, showed that chronic stress depletes our adrenal glands and impairs our ability to respond to immune challenges such as infections or cancer. Acute stress stimulates our ability to react, but long-standing and recurrent stress exhausts our immune system. The following case is not unusual:

> After being passed over for a promotion a year ago, Donald knew he was in a dead-end job. Sensing that he was never going to realize the professional and financial goals he had set for himself, Donald was emotionally and physically exhausted. He tried unsuccessfully to boost his depleted energy with innumerable cups of strong coffee throughout the day. Despite his ongoing fatigue, he was unable to sleep at night, so he resorted to downing several shots of bourbon before bed. He also began smoking again, even though he didn't really enjoy the habit anymore. His relationship with his wife deteriorated to the point that they were barely on speaking terms.
>
> When his stomach began cramping, he assumed his ulcer was acting up again. After unsuccessfully treating himself with over-the-counter remedies for several months, he sought help from his gastroenterologist. His doctor performed a study to look at his stomach and took a few biopsy specimens from an active irritation. To the surprise of both Donald and his doctor, one of the biopsy brushings returned positive for stomach cancer.

Let's speculate on the dialogue between mind and body that contributes to this situation. Our brains are continuously transmitting information on our emotional state to our body through a number of chemical messengers called neurotransmitters. We used to think that these transmitter molecules were only used for one nerve cell to speak to another, but we now know that many cells in our body can receive and understand these chemical communications. Among the most important cells listening to our mental conversation are those of our immune system. The conversation may sound like this:

DONALD'S MIND: I can't believe I didn't get my promotion. . . . Now, I'll never advance in this organization. . . . It looks like I'll be forever stuck in this crummy job. . . . I can't stand this depressed feeling. . . . I think I'll numb my pain with a few shots of Johnny Walker Red.

DONALD'S BRAIN: I'm not in the mood to make any pleasure chemicals, and I'm not receiving any messages to create energy-enhancing molecules. . . . I think I'll go into partial shutdown for a while until Donald figures out his next move.

DONALD'S IMMUNE CELLS: These are very depressing chemical messages I'm receiving. . . . I don't feel particularly aggressive about that funny-looking stomach cell. . . . I'll let one of the other guys deal with it.

Although this scenario is an oversimplification, there is good evidence to support that our negative mental states impair our immune function, while our positive states enhance it. If you've had a stressful month, you are more likely to get the symptoms of a cold when exposed to a virus than if your life was pretty relaxed.[2] If you are facing a final examination and are not sure you're adequately prepared, your immune cells may not be at peak performance.[3] On a more serious note, if you have recently been divorced or lost a spouse, your natural killer cells function in a depressed manner corresponding to your grief.[4]

One of the most fascinating studies that demonstrate how our interpretations can influence our immune system was performed over twenty years ago at the University of Rochester by Dr. Robert Ader.[5] Although his experiment was performed in rats, it offers remarkable insights into how our minds can affect our physical health. In this study, rats were given injections of the potent chemotherapy drug cyclophosphamide just as they tasted water that was sweetened with saccharin. One of the immediate side effects of this drug is nausea, so giving this injection to rats promptly induced vomiting. Because cyclophosphamide is also a powerful immune suppressant, the rats that received it showed weakening of their immune systems for several days after the injection.

Once their immune systems had recovered, Dr. Ader repeated the experiment, but this time when the rats tasted the saccharin-sweetened water, he gave them an injection of salt water. Because they had been conditioned to associate the sweetened water with nausea, they again

promptly vomited upon tasting the sweetness. This was a classical example of neuro-associative conditioning. In the same way that Pavlov had
conditioned dogs to salivate when he rang a bell, because they had previously associated the sound with the offering of food, these rats were
conditioned to vomit when they tasted sweetened water. What was as-
tonishing in the second part of Ader's experiment was the finding that the
rats showed suppression in their immune function despite the fact that no
active drug was given. Their immune cells had "learned" that sweetened
water caused them to be suppressed. Merely the perception and interpretation of sweet water as a stress created a profound physiological effect
that meant the difference between sickness and health.

This amazing finding that immune cells can learn has widespread
implications. Other studies have shown that many people who undergo
chemotherapy treatment for cancer begin to feel nauseated on their way
to the next treatment visit and show signs of immune suppression even
before they receive the next course of medicine. These responses are
known as anticipated nausea and vomiting (ANV) and anticipated immune suppression (AIS).[6] As I will be discussing in detail in chapter 6, I
believe there are ways we can transform this negative learning into a positive response by creating nourishing, stress-reducing associations, rather
than the typical anxiety-provoking ones.

The Stress of Life

All stress is ultimately related to loss or the fear of loss. With ongoing
stress, our immune system runs down, and when our immune system is
weary, we are more vulnerable to a number of illnesses, including cancer.
The worst stress occurs when we are facing a circumstance over which we
feel that we have little or no control. This is true whether we're talking
about laboratory mice subjected to stress in a cage or the Shah of Iran
watching his country going through a fundamentalist revolution to which
he was not invited. Uncertainty is a fact of life that offers the possibility
for both joy and sorrow. When we unexpectedly fall in love, receive a
promotion, or encounter an old school friend, we appreciate the uncertainty for the pleasure it brings. When, on the other hand, we discover a
lover has been unfaithful, are fired from a job, or learn that a family member is ill, the uncertainty brings anxiety and a sense of being out of control. At these times we are more vulnerable to illness, and the longer our
sense of vulnerability lasts, the more our immunity is compromised.

It's naive, however, to suggest that there is a simple correlation between stress and cancer. Life is too elusive to be pinned down that easily.
This is why humility is so important in this area. We have all seen people experiencing overwhelming stress who do not develop cancer. Similarly, it is not uncommon for me to see sick people whose illnesses defy
explanation.

> Janet was really ready to enjoy her life. Her two children were
> thriving in school, her husband was happy at his job, and she was
> registered for a creative writing class at the community college.
> She had always been careful about her diet, never smoked, and
> rarely drank alcohol. She had just started yoga and exercise
> classes and looked forward to greater flexibility and fitness. Janet
> was initially unconcerned about the little lump she noticed in her
> neck above her breastbone, but she mentioned it to her doctor
> when she went in for a routine examination. He described it as a
> nodule in her thyroid and recommended a needle biopsy. It was
> quite a blow when she received his call a few days later telling her
> the report showed papillary thyroid cancer.
>
> The next six months were challenging as she underwent
> more extensive surgery and radioactive iodine treatment, but
> by her last exam, all evidence of cancer was gone. When asked
> what meaning this illness had for her, she responded that it
> symbolized her prior lack of willingness to express herself. She
> related that she had always placed others' needs ahead of her
> own and became aware of suppressed anger during her illness.
> Her bout with cancer has given her permission to fulfill her
> own needs and express her feelings to family and friends. To
> her joy and delight, her husband and children truly appreciate
> her more powerful nature and fully support her desire to ex-
> press her creativity. She now looks back on her experience with
> gratitude.

When a heavy smoker develops throat cancer, we may not question
why his illness arose. When someone like Janet gets sick, our sense of
order is threatened, and we search, often unsuccessfully, for some reasonable explanation. But, even if we cannot easily understand why someone's
mind-body system allows cancer to arise, we can at any moment make
choices to strengthen our immunity and improve our overall quality of
life. By choosing behaviors that bring us joy and comfort in *this* moment,
we can generate a healing mind-body environment that promotes health.

When our mind experiences pleasure, our brain releases healing chemicals. We can think of this as our immune cells perpetually eavesdropping on our internal conversation.

Enlivening Our Immunity

Whether you can identify a significant stress in your life preceding the onset of cancer, learning you have a serious illness is a universally stressful experience. This is when your choices can make a real impact on how you deal with the cancer threat. Just as we know that stress weakens our immune function, we have learned that nurturing experiences can strengthen our immunity. In this book we'll be covering many simple approaches for improving the quality of information that flows between our mind and our body. Meditation techniques that quiet the mind, nutritional choices that nurture the body, emotional clearing processes that replace self-destructive feelings with life-affirming ones, and simple sensory nourishing techniques can all be used to enliven our deepest healing potential.

Although we are just beginning to understand *why* these mind-body approaches can be valuable, there is increasingly abundant information to support their efficacy. Dr. Carl Simonton was a pioneer in mind-body approaches for cancer, popularizing visualization techniques in which patients imagined their immune cells gobbling up malignant ones. Although he did not conduct controlled studies, he reported exceptional outcomes in many patients with cancer who actively envisioned healing images.[7]

Psychiatrist Dr. David Spiegel of Stanford University had been developing support groups for people with cancer for a number of years, finding that patients' life quality improved when they expressed their concerns in a nurturing environment. Using the combination of group support and relaxation techniques, his patients experienced less pain, less anxiety, more energy, and better sleeping patterns.[8] Based on these positive experiences, he analyzed whether these mind-body approaches improved the quantity as well as the quality of life for these women with breast cancer. To his astonishment, the women participating in the support group not only felt better; they lived almost twice as long as those receiving standard cancer care.[9]

Dr. Fawzy Fawzy at UCLA found similar results in his patients with a malignant melanoma, a form of skin cancer. Those who participated in a six-week mind-body program experienced healthier moods, healthier immune function, and longer survival.[10] While these programs are very inspiring to people with cancer, it is a commentary on our current health system that despite documented benefit, cancer support groups are not considered standard care in most health institutions. If a medication were found to double the survival time in people with cancer, it would be considered malpractice not to offer it. Unfortunately, our medical system is so pharmacologically oriented that in most communities, lay support groups are organized outside of institutional cancer centers. This is slowly changing as health care systems begin to recognize that mind-body programs not only enhance the care of people with cancer but can also be cost-effective.

Changing the Message

When people with cancer ask for our help at the Chopra Center, we tell them we do not treat cancer. As far as I am aware, none of the approaches we offer has a direct effect on cancer cells in the same way that chemotherapy or radiation does. Although certain herbs have anticancer effects, most of these studies have been on cells cultured in test tubes, not on real people with cancer.

We do believe that our programs treat people with cancer. By this I mean that we are dedicated to improving a person's quality of life by reconnecting body, mind, and spirit. I spoke earlier in this chapter about fear and its harmful effect on our health. According to Vedic science, all fear is quantified fear of mortality. As long as our sense of self is identified with material things—our positions and possessions—we will experience fear as a prevailing emotion. This includes identification with our physical body. The nature of the world of name and form that we perceive through our senses is that it is always changing. Change is synonymous with uncertainty, and uncertainty is uncomfortable, for every change implies some loss. The only way to overcome fear is to get in touch with something that is beyond change. And the only thing beyond change is the field of intelligence, of spirit, that is at the basis of change.

The goal of *Return to Wholeness* is to remind you of your essential nature, which is timeless and boundless. It is also fearless, because when spirit is our internal reference point we cannot entertain the possibility of loss. Contact with this aspect of ourselves is the basis of healing. Just a taste of immortality can vanquish our anxiety and open the possibility for profound transformation. All techniques of healing have their most powerful impact when they remind us of our true essence as aspects of a greater whole. Meditation that takes us to an expanded state of inner awareness, healthy nutrition that connects us with our environment, sensory techniques that enliven our mind-body connection, and loving social support that reminds us that we are not alone—all these approaches can be viewed as restorers of wholeness. When we are reminded of our oneness with life, we transcend our fear and gain immunity from suffering. Let's learn some ways to part the veil of fear.

Commitment to Wholeness

Our bodies are the end products of our experiences and interpretations. To change our bodies, we need to change our experiences. Make a commitment to change your life in the direction of greater love and caring for yourself and those close to you.

1. I consciously choose to spend some time in silence each day, connecting with my quiet self. When I am feeling caught up in my fears and anxieties, I will seek comfort in family and friends who remind me that I am loved and not alone.

2. I commit to spending some time enjoying myself every day. It may be a walk in the park, getting a massage, or playing with my pets. I will do something each day that has no value other than making me happy.

3. When I catch myself ruminating over distressing thoughts, I will change my activity by listening to some enjoyable music, dancing, going for a walk, or reading a good book.

CHAPTER 3

Nutritional Healing

Food for Nourishment, Balance, and Joy

When we develop reverence for food and the miracle of transformation
inherent in it, just the simple act of eating creates a ritual of celebration.
—DEEPAK CHOPRA

Eating was never a great source of pleasure for Laura. Her childhood mealtimes were chaotic, and she recalls being compelled to
eat even when she was not hungry. As an adult, she rarely prepared a home-cooked meal, usually consuming fast foods on the
run. She was always quite thin, occasionally prompting friends to
ask her if she had an eating disorder.

Her relationship to food changed when she developed cancer
of the cervix. A routine Pap smear showed localized cancer cells
requiring an operation that fortunately removed all the malignant tissue. However, the shock of facing a serious illness jolted
her into looking at the basics of her life. She began eating healthier foods, taking cooking classes, and studying nutrition. She
gained some well-needed weight and noticed that her energy
level improved. More important, Laura realized that eating could
be an enjoyable experience. For the first time in her life, she
started believing that she truly deserved to be nourished.

Next to breathing, eating is our most primordial action. We seek
nourishment from our environment as soon as we are born, and spend a
good part of the rest of our lives thinking about and consuming food. As
the rarely disputed pinnacle of the terrestrial food chain, we are capable
of devouring a vast array of animal and vegetable species, although each

human culture labels a limited number of ingestibles as truly edible. Food shapes our physical, emotional, and spiritual vision of ourselves. The types of foods we place in our mouths identify our place in the world as much as our religion, nationality, or political convictions. It may be a cliché, but it is nonetheless true, that we are what we eat.

Each of us is a localized network of intelligence in the vast field of energy and information we call the universe. Through our senses we ingest the sounds, sensations, sights, and smells of the information-rich world around us, and the most tangible way we receive the energy of our environment is through the food we eat. We consume the biological intelligence of plants and animals and convert it into the energy and information of our body. Although living beings have been performing this alchemy since the beginning of life, we have as human beings added unprecedented layers of complexity to this primordial process. It's my goal in this chapter to restore the ease and simplicity that eating deserves. Recapturing the natural joyfulness of eating is particularly important if you are facing a serious illness such as cancer.

Three basic components of eating are necessary to create and maintain a healthy physiology: our food must be nourishing, our digestive power should be strong, and our elimination should be efficient. If any one of these three is less than ideal, the possibility of disease arises. How do we know whether food is nourishing? It's not an easy question to answer. As Lucretius once said, "One man's poison is another man's food." Most Americans do not relish termite grubs, and only the boldest among us delight in the slimy taste of raw sea urchin, but this doesn't stop people of other cultures from prizing these treats as delicious delicacies. Although traditional food choices in a culture persist across generations, the emergence of our global village is exposing large segments of earth's population to expanded nutritional options. In America, we show a remarkable flexibility in shifting our culinary preferences as a result of new information that nutritional science presents to us on a regular basis.

The standard meat-and-potatoes diet of the fifties reflected an emphasis on abundant protein, considered essential for building strong tissues. With the rise of heart disease and its association with animal fat, nutritional experts began recommending less red meat. As our understanding of the relationship between food and health deepens, we are seeing a new awareness of nutrition and its role in individual, societal, and ecological well being.

This new scrutiny of food has also brought unnecessary stress and confusion to our most basic of behaviors. I commonly see people who have received so many different opinions about what and what not to eat that they are literally afraid of food. The idea that eating is meant to be enjoyable—a true celebration of life—needs to be reintroduced into our understanding of nutrition. If I am following the "diet of the month" but not savoring the experience of eating, I am not really nourishing myself.

Several times each year, a new book promoting a novel nutritional program reaches the best-seller list, promising to improve your health, help you lose weight, and give you more energy. Many of these approaches are valid, but they inevitably fade into history for several simple reasons. First, many of the popular designer diet programs are unnatural. With constant attention, we may be able to follow a plan that precisely regulates nutritional components, but most of us quickly tire of the need for such nonstop control. It is also challenging for most people to maintain their enthusiasm for the various liquid or powdered supplements often recommended to gain the benefits of some programs. Second, most of the restrictive diets are not very delicious. We can muster some discipline for a dietary regimen if we feel it will bring us long-term benefit, but if our basic need for appetizing tastes is not met, it's unlikely that we will stay with a program for long. Finally, most dietary programs do not recognize that one size does not fit all. People are put together differently, and a diet that may be appropriate for one person may actually be harmful for another. For a diet to be beneficial and practical, it should be natural, delicious, and flexible enough for people with diverse needs to enjoy it.

The Major Players— Carbohydrates, Protein, Fats, and Fiber

The nutritional energy of nature is available to us in the form of three major categories: carbohydrates, proteins, and fats. Fiber benefits us because it cannot be digested. I'll briefly review what is known about these common foodstuffs and cancer and then offer my suggestions for a health-enhancing diet.

1. Carbohydrates. Breads, pasta, rice, grains, and sugar comprise the bulk of the carbohydrates we consume. Our consumption of carbohydrates is only half as much as that eaten by a typical American at the beginning of the twentieth century. We have substituted fats and protein for the whole grains that were once the staple of our diet. In general, we could

benefit from increasing our total intake of carbohydrates to 55 percent from our current average 45 percent, by eating more whole grain breads, pastas, starchy vegetables, and beans, *not* by eating more refined sugars. In addition to providing a ready energy source, these complex carbohydrates are also high in fiber. With regard to cancer, excessive carbohydrate intake is a concern only as it contributes to obesity, which is a risk factor for breast and uterine cancer. Higher intake of refined and processed dietary sugar has been associated with slightly increased risks of breast and colon cancer, but not enough to make you feel guilty about an occasional chocolate chip cookie.

2. Protein. Protein is essential to good health, but many nutritional experts now believe that we have been consuming excessive amounts. A minimal protein intake of about 5 percent of our daily calories is necessary for good health and growth. This works out to about thirty grams per day, which is contained in about four ounces of meat, fish, or poultry or about four glasses of milk. Children, pregnant women, and strenuously active men need more, primarily to ensure that they are receiving the essential amino acids that are necessary for building healthy tissues. Plant sources such as beans, nuts, and grains provide high-quality protein, but must be combined to guarantee that all the essential amino acid building blocks are present.

High levels of protein have been associated with higher rates of a variety of cancers, including breast, pancreatic, prostate, and colon cancer.[1] It seems that the relationship between protein and cancer is mainly due to excesses in animal protein, which is almost always linked with higher levels of saturated fat. It's safe to say that most Americans' health would benefit from reducing their intake of animal protein.

3. Fat. The fat in our diet has received a lot of attention as a risk factor for heart disease. It's now clear that too much fat, particularly animal fat, also raises our risk for cancer. Breast, prostate, and colon cancers are much more common in societies like ours, which consume a lot of fat.

Why fat increases our cancer risk is less clear. There are several possible explanations for this:[2]

~ Fats may be digested into potential cancer-causing chemicals.
~ Fats may carry carcinogens from the environment into our bodies.
~ Fats may change the way we metabolize hormones.
~ Fats may alter our immune systems.

Regardless of why too much fat raises our risk of cancer, it is clear that reducing our intake can benefit our health. It is easy to accomplish this by simply reducing our consumption of animal products. If you are eating red meat on a regular basis, make the choice to reduce your intake in half, substituting fish, fowl, and vegetarian entrées for that steak or hamburger. Your body and the environment will thank you.

4. Fiber. More than twenty-five years ago studies suggested that people who ate more plants had less cancer, in part due to the abundance of vegetable fiber. Plant fiber is mainly found in cell walls, where it keeps the cell from bursting or collapsing. Since we don't have enzymes to digest it, fiber increases our elimination bulk. Fiber may dilute carcinogens we have ingested, bind them so they are not absorbed, or change the bacteria in our colon so they are not converted into active cancer-causing chemicals. Although we don't fully understand why, most nutritional experts believe that eating high-fiber foods is beneficial.[3] Bran, whole grain breads, brown rice, apples, berries, pitted fruits, beans, and most vegetables are high in fiber and should be a substantial part of every diet. However, if you are not accustomed to a high-fiber diet and have tumors in your abdomen, be sure to check with your physician before making a dietary shift.

Eating Naturally, Eating Wisely

The American Cancer Society has made some simple recommendations to reduce the risk of cancer, suggesting seven dietary guidelines:

1. Avoid obesity.
2. Eat a varied diet.
3. Include a variety of vegetables and fruits.
4. Eat more high-fiber foods.
5. Cut down on total fat intake.
6. Eat fewer smoked, salted, and nitrite-cured foods.
7. Limit alcohol consumption.

These principles seem so simple and yet the incidence of cancer continues to rise in our society. How do we translate these simple principles into a dietary program that is inspiring and nourishing? These recommendations have been promoted for a number of years, and we may be seeing a shift in our culture's nutritional choices, but many people fear that they have to make a choice between eating for health or eating for enjoyment. This is where the nutritional principles of Ayurveda offer great value. They provide approaches that are balanced, natural, enjoyable, specific, and delicious. Ayurveda is a vast ocean of information that offers nutritional advice to promote health, even if you are facing a serious illness. The nutritional wisdom of Ayurveda expands and complements the practical advice that modern nutrition provides.

Science of Life Nutrition

The seers of Ayurveda were true scientists. Although they were not armed with microscopes or MRI units, they were careful observers of the world, describing the influence of foods, herbs, sounds, smells, and sensations on human beings in health and illness. The principles of Ayurvedic nutrition continue to amaze and fascinate me, for they remain relevant five thousand years after they were codified. The Ayurvedic classification of food into practical categories enables us to make healthy choices even without a Ph.D. in nutritional science. Let's explore some of these basic principles.

The Tastes of Life

Modern nutritional science recognizes four tastes—sweet, sour, salty, and bitter. Ayurveda adds two more—pungent and astringent, which can be perceived as sensations on the tongue more than actual tastes. According to Ayurvedic lore, nature packages all possible food sources into one or more of these six tastes so we know which foods are nourishing and how much to consume. All six tastes should be eaten at every meal for us to feel satisfied and to ensure that all major food groups and nutrients are represented. Let's review them.

Sweet taste is the flavor of foods that promote growth and regeneration. Because our tissues are classified as sweet, foods that carry this taste increase the bulk of our body. Sweet applies not only to refined sugars that should be limited in any healthy diet, but also includes carbohydrates, protein, and fats. Whether we are growing children or recovering from a debilitating illness, sweet foods should be abundant in our diet. The most common foods that are considered sweet in Ayurveda are milk, rice, pasta, breads, nuts, sweet fruits, and starchy vegetables such as potatoes, yams, and corn.

Sour taste comes from organic acids like those found in citrus fruits, berries, tomatoes, and vinegar. Yogurt and buttermilk are also predominantly sour in taste. The sour taste stimulates salivation and kindles our appetite. It is a very useful taste when hunger is suppressed, as it is during chemotherapy treatments. Foods with sour taste also dispel intestinal gas and help to reduce bloating when your bowels are sluggish. A regular dose of foods with the sour taste ensures among other things that we are receiving adequate vitamin C.

The *salty* taste is found in mineral salts, either in the form of rock salt or sea salt. Salt stimulates the appetite, enhances digestion, and is both mildly laxative and mildly sedative. Water follows salt in the body so that excessive salt intake leads to fluid retention, but a little bit of salt can make the difference between a dish's being bland or tasty. In addition to crystalline salt, tamari, soy sauce, and kelp are used commonly in Asian countries to supply this taste.

Pungent taste is the hot sensation found in peppers and aromatic spices. It is carried by essential oils that have the effect of sharpening the appetite and stimulating digestion. Pungent substances include black pepper, horseradish, cayenne, ginger, peppermint, garlic, cinnamon, and mustard. Studies on essential oils derived from spicy plants such as garlic, onion, and horseradish have shown they contain potent antioxidant substances that are capable of deactivating potential cancer-causing chemicals.[4, 5] Most of us have experienced the direct effect of pungent foods when we accidentally bite into a jalapeño pepper and begin sweating. These heat-containing substances can also be used therapeutically to relieve nasal congestion. Americans tend to be shy about the spicy taste, but gourmets from Mexico, Asia, and the Middle East prize spices that add heat to a meal.

Bitter taste alone is not very appealing but has the value of enlivening our other tastes. It is detoxifying and cooling to the system. Bitter flavor is due to a food's content of alkaloid or glycoside chemicals. Most green and yellow vegetables have some degree of bitterness, with green leafy vegetables having the highest content of naturally bitter chemicals. Asparagus, broccoli, carrots, celery, chard, green peppers, spinach, lettuce, and kale all carry the bitter taste. Many of the culinary and medicinal herbs are predominantly bitter. The bitter taste of vegetables and herbs may reflect their content of substances called phytochemicals, which are powerful natural cancer-fighting agents. I'll be discussing them in greater detail in another chapter.

Astringent taste is more of a sensation than a flavor. It's the sensation that makes your mouth pucker. Astringency is due to a food's content of tannins, which have a drying effect on mucous membranes and a toning and compacting effect on tissues. Many common nutritional sources have some astringent qualities, including tea, honey, walnuts, and pomegranates. Dried beans, lentils, and peas are also considered to have an astringent component, providing a valuable source of protein and carbohydrate. Many vegetables are both bitter and astringent, like broccoli, celery, lettuce, and spinach. Grains like rye, whole wheat, and couscous and some fruits, including apples, berries, figs, and lemons, carry the astringent taste along with other flavors. Recent studies have suggested that chemicals in tea may reduce the risk of a number of cancers, including those of the digestive and urinary tracts. Even decaffeinated teas may have a similar protective effect.[6, 7] I predict that in coming years we will be learning a lot more about the health benefits of the natural chemicals that comprise astringent foods.

Making Eating Simple

If you eat foods representing each of the six taste categories at every meal, you will have a nutritionally balanced, health-promoting, and delicious diet. Let's see what this might look like.

Breakfast

Orange juice (sweet, sour)
Hot cream of wheat cereal with blueberries (sweet, astringent)
Low-fat milk (sweet)
Egg-white vegetable omelet with onions, peppers, zucchini, and tomatoes, seasoned with oregano, basil, dill, and salt herbs and spices (sweet, pungent, sour, bitter, salty)
A cup of tea (astringent)

Lunch

Linguini with low-fat pesto made from spinach, cilantro, fresh basil, lemon juice, and pine nuts (sweet, sour, salty, bitter, pungent, astringent)
Grated Parmesan cheese (sweet, sour, salty)
Spinach salad with mandarin oranges and light oil and vinegar dressing (astringent, sour)
Steamed zucchini with cumin (bitter, pungent)
Baked apple with maple syrup (sweet, astringent)

Dinner

Lentil soup with carrots, onions, and spices (astringent, sweet, pungent, salty)
Wild rice with raisins (sweet, astringent)
Baked multigrain bread with clarified butter (sweet)
Asparagus spears with grated almonds (bitter, sweet)
Fresh strawberries with honey and yogurt (sour, sweet, astringent)

I hope you'll agree that a nutritional program that puts into practice the principles outlined above can be both balanced and delicious. In addition to fully satisfying your taste buds, a meal plan based upon the six tastes more than satisfies the American Cancer Society's recommendations for consuming five or more servings of fruits and vegetables each day. If you are not prepared to forsake all sources of animal protein, you could easily add seafood to the linguini for lunch or chicken to the lentil soup. Each meal scores high in antioxidant-rich vegetables and fruits, low in fat, and high in fiber. When all six tastes are represented, you will feel satisfied when you're finished eating.

Food as Medicine

In addition to serving as a source of nutrition, food can help balance mind and body. According to Ayurveda, there are three dynamic principles at work in our physiology: movement, metabolism, and structure. Metaphorically, they can be thought of as the forces of wind, fire, and earth. These primary forces are influenced by everything we ingest through our five senses, including the food we eat. The movement, or "Wind," principle governs the action of thought, respiration, circulation, and digestion. The metabolism, or "Fire," principle governs the digestion of food, mental discrimination, temperature regulation, and inflammatory responses in our body. The structure, or "Earth," principle lubricates our respiratory tract, digestive system, and joints and governs the regulation of water and fat. It also stabilizes our mind.

When these three basic principles are in harmony, the right balance of dynamism, transformation, and stability supports our well being. During every illness, however, these basic forces become unbalanced and result in distressing symptoms. Too much wind manifests itself as anxiety, insomnia, digestive irritability, and constipation. Too much fire shows up

	Characteristic of me . . .				
	Not at all	Slightly	Some-what	Moder-ately	Very
1. I have been feeling anxious.	1	2	3	4	5
2. I have been having trouble sleeping.	1	2	3	4	5
3. My appetite has been weak.	1	2	3	4	5
4. I have been constipated.	1	2	3	4	5
5. I have lost more than five pounds.	1	2	3	4	5
6. My skin has been dry or flaky.	1	2	3	4	5
7. My eating and sleeping schedule has been erratic.	1	2	3	4	5
8. My hands and feet have been cold.	1	2	3	4	5
9. I have had a lot of intestinal gas.	1	2	3	4	5
10. I have a dry, nonproductive cough.	1	2	3	4	5

Total for Section 1 = Movement ("Wind") _____

	Not at all	Slightly	Some-what	Moder-ately	Very
1. I have been irritable.	1	2	3	4	5
2. I have been losing my temper.	1	2	3	4	5
3. I have been overheated or having hot flashes.	1	2	3	4	5
4. I have been having heartburn.	1	2	3	4	5
5. I have had burning with urination or defecation.	1	2	3	4	5
6. I regularly have more than two bowel movements per day.	1	2	3	4	5
7. I have been breaking out with skin rashes.	1	2	3	4	5
8. My tongue or mouth have been raw or sore.	1	2	3	4	5
9. I have been having burning pain.	1	2	3	4	5
10. I have been having a strong body smell.	1	2	3	4	5

Total for Section 2 = Metabolism ("Fire") _____

	Characteristic of me . . .				
	Not at all	Slightly	Some-what	Moder-ately	Very
1. I have been sleeping a lot.	1	2	3	4	5
2. I have been retaining fluid.	1	2	3	4	5
3. I have been having nasal congestion.	1	2	3	4	5
4. I have gained more than five pounds.	1	2	3	4	5
5. I have a wet, productive cough.	1	2	3	4	5
6. My joints are swollen.	1	2	3	4	5
7. My thinking has been slow.	1	2	3	4	5
8. I feel heavy and dull after eating.	1	2	3	4	5
9. I have been feeling nauseated.	1	2	3	4	5
10. I have been feeling emotionally withdrawn.	1	2	3	4	5
Total for Section 3 = Structure ("Earth")					

as indigestion, fever, and irritability. Too much earth is expressed as lethargy, congestion, and fluid retention. By knowing which of our basic mind-body principles is off balance, we can make choices that reestablish our equilibrium.

To learn about your current mind-body status according to Ayurvedic principles, please complete the questionnaire on pages 46–47. Using the scale, indicate how well each statement applies to your life experiences over the past thirty to sixty days.

Your highest-scoring mind-body principle is the one that usually needs the most attention. Any score above 30 points also suggests the need for balancing. Wind, earth, and fire can be balanced through each of the senses and the foods we eat.

Wind

Due to her polycystic ovary syndrome, Alison had always had irregular menstrual periods, but when she continued bleeding for several weeks, her gynecologist recommended a dilatation and curettage (D & C). The pathology report returned positive for endometrial cancer, and although her surgeon expressed confidence that her treatment would be successful, she became increasingly anxious. She awakened several times each night with her mind racing, her digestion became very delicate, and she was troubled by constipation. She could barely force herself to eat and was losing weight. She knew she needed to ground herself before proceeding with the recommended surgery, so she learned meditation and began following a "Wind" pacifying program. She focused on eating warm, simple foods, taking a warm bath with ginger powder, and drinking hot milk with nutmeg before bed and getting regular calming massages. She was soon sleeping better at night and feeling more settled. She got through her surgery without complications and continues to follow many of the same calming rituals simply because they make her feel better, even through she no longer worries about cancer.

If your "Wind" score is high, you are probably experiencing a feeling of being ungrounded. Warm and heavy foods and those with sweet, sour, and salty tastes are grounding and include whole grain breads, pasta, rice, hearty vegetable soups, nuts, honey, warm milk, and sweet fruits. Particularly if you are feeling debilitated from your illness, increasing your intake of these nourishing foods will help you gain weight and restore your energy.

Fire

Since the excision of the malignant mole from his shoulder, Michael had been very irritable. Although he had always been somewhat of a perfectionist, he became excessively compulsive about his business, often staying up until two in the morning to catch up on work he had missed due to his surgery. His indigestion was worse, and he was having three or more bowel movements each day. His temper flared easily, and employees and family members felt they had to walk on eggshells around him to avoid "awakening the dragon."

Michael started a "Fire"-reducing program that included foods that were cooling. He was encouraged to express his mortality fears and to take some playtime each day. A couple of months later he told me he just needed to stop taking himself so seriously. Soon after his visit with us, his heartburn cooled down, and the people in his life felt it was safe to be around him again.

If your "Fire" score is elevated, you are probably feeling hot and irritable. To reduce the heat in your body, reduce your intake of spicy, sour, and salty foods and increase those with sweet, bitter, and astringent tastes. Milk products, breads, lentils, white rice, potatoes, cucumbers, and sweet fruits are cooling to the system. Throughout this book we'll be discussing how to use all the senses to cool off a raging metabolism.

Earth

Michelle was tolerating her Hodgkin's disease treatment fairly well except for some fluid retention and tiredness. She had always tended to be overweight, and the steroids she was taking as part of her chemotherapy contributed to her sense of heaviness and congestion. She was placed on an "Earth"-lightening program, including lighter foods with pungent, bitter, and astringent tastes. She was encouraged to get to bed by ten at night and be up by seven in the morning. With this program she was able to complete her treatment protocol, noticing that much of her lethargy and heaviness resolved.

If your "Earth" score is excessive, you are probably feeling sluggish, heavy, and congested. To create greater lightness and flexibility eat foods that are warm, light, and dry, favoring pungent, bitter, and astringent

Mind-Body Principle	Wind	Fire	Earth
Signs of imbalance	Anxiety, insomnia, delicate digestion, constipation	Irritability, diarrhea, hot flashes, skin rashes	Lethargy, weight gain, fluid retention, congestion
Tastes to favor	Sweet, sour, salty	Sweet, bitter, astringent	Pungent, bitter, astringent
Foods to favor	Dairy, starchy vegetables, sweet fruits, nuts	Milk, whole grains, rice, corn, sweet fruits	Green leafy vegetables, apples, pears, tofu
Spices to favor	Pepper, ginger, cinnamon, salt, mustard	Mint, cardamom, cumin, fennel, cilantro	Basil, pepper, ginger, cloves, nutmeg
Sweeteners to favor	Honey, fructose, maple syrup	Raw sugar, fructose	Honey

	To pacify "Wind"	To pacify "Fire"	To pacify "Earth"
	favor	*favor*	*favor*
	Warm, oily, heavy foods	*Cool foods and liquids*	*Light, dry, warm foods*
	Sweet, sour, salty tastes	*Sweet, bitter,*	*Pungent, bitter,*
		astringent tastes	*astringent tastes*
DAIRY	Favor: all dairy	Favor: milk, butter, ghee	Favor: low-fat milk
		Reduce: yogurt, cheese, sour cream	Reduce: all other dairy
FRUITS	Favor: avocados, bananas, cherries, mangos	Favor: grapes, melons, cherries, apples, ripe oranges	Favor: apples, pears
	Reduce: apples, pears, cranberries	Reduce: grapefruits, sour berries	Reduce: bananas, avocados, coconuts, melons
VEGE-TABLES	Favor: asparagus, beets, carrots	Favor: asparagus, cucumbers, potatoes, broccoli, green beans	Favor: all vegetables except tomatoes, cucumbers, sweet potatoes
	Reduce: sprouts, cabbage	Reduce: tomatoes, peppers, onions, radishes	
BEANS	Favor: mung and tofu	Favor: all beans except lentils	Favor: all beans except tofu and soybeans
	Reduce: all other beans		
GRAINS	Favor: rice and wheat	Favor: rice, wheat, barley, oats	Favor: barley, corn, millet, buckwheat, rye, oats
	Reduce: barley, corn, millet, buckwheat, rye, oats	Reduce: corn, millet, brown rice	Reduce: rice and wheat
SWEET-ENERS	Favor: all sweeteners	Favor: all sweeteners except molasses	Favor: honey
			Reduce: all other sweeteners
OILS	Favor: all oils	Favor: olive, sunflower, coconut	Favor: almond, sunflower in small quantities
		Reduce: sesame, almond, corn	Reduce: all others
SPICES	Favor: cardamom, cumin, ginger, cinnamon, salt, cloves, mustard seed, black pepper	Favor: coriander, cumin, fennel	Favor: all spices
		Reduce: hot spices like ginger, pepper, mustard seed	Reduce: salt

tastes. Corn, barley, and millet eaten in combination with split peas, lentils, and tofu will ensure complete protein with minimal fat. Dairy products should be nonfat, and most sweeteners should be minimized, although a little honey is acceptable. Most spices, especially those that are pungent such as pepper, ginger, cumin, and mustard, are useful in mobilizing secretions and reducing congestion.

Purifying and Rejuvenating Foods

Facing cancer is always stressful, and when under stress, both our minds and our bodies tend to accumulate toxicity. Our anxious thoughts and feelings of depression may create more distress than the actual malignancy we are facing. Physically, cancer and the powerful therapies to treat it take their toll on our digestion, bowel habits, sleep patterns, and energy level. This accumulated toxicity expresses itself as a number of psychological and physical symptoms:

~ Fatigue
~ Irritability
~ Lack of alertness
~ Coated tongue
~ Depression
~ Generalized aching
~ Loss of appetite
~ Unpleasant body odor
~ Indigestion
~ Sour taste
~ Weakness
~ Loss of taste
~ Joint pain
~ Heaviness
~ Bad breath

When these symptoms are present, favoring a diet that is lighter and easier to digest can help reduce accumulated toxicity. There are a number of dietary recommendations that can facilitate the detoxification process:

~ All food should be freshly prepared. Minimize canned, frozen, and leftover foods.
~ Eat lighter foods such as vegetable soups, lentil, and rice.

~   Favor freshly steamed or lightly sautéed vegetables.
~   Reduce heavy dairy products such as aged cheeses and sour cream.
~   Eliminate alcohol.
~   Reduce your intake of saturated fats and oils.
~   Reduce your intake of refined sugars.
~   If you cannot eliminate animal products, favor seafood and the white meat of turkey and chicken. Minimize beef and pork.

In addition to ensuring that the food we consume is nutritious and easy to digest, there are simple things we can do to enhance our digestive power. If your appetite has been weak and you have had to force yourself to eat, try stimulating your hunger with bitter and pungent herbs and spices. Bitter tonics like gentian, golden seal, and barberry have been used as medicinal substances in the West for generations. They stimulate stomach emptying and clear our taste buds. Readily available bitter herbs include turmeric, coriander, and dill. Pungent herbs help to stimulate digestion and are best taken five or ten minutes before your meal. A delicious apéritif that we use at the Chopra Center consists of equal parts gingerroot juice, lemon juice, honey, and water with a pinch of black pepper. An ounce before a meal can enliven your appetite and digestion.

Liquid fasting is another way to help detoxify the body. Consuming only fresh-squeezed juices from fruits and vegetables for a day can create lightness and kindle digestive power. Citrus fruits, apples, pears, and grapes make great and easily obtainable juices. Vegetables that can be juiced include carrots, beets, cucumber, and spinach. If you are carrying extra weight, you can follow a juice diet one day a week. If you are having trouble maintaining your weight, a liquid diet should be used sparingly. Perhaps one or two days a month try drinking juices for breakfast and lunch and then having some soup or steamed vegetables for dinner. It's best to reduce your activity level on the day that you are juicing so as not to overtax your body.

Replenishing Foods

Loss of appetite and loss of weight are common in people facing cancer. Both cancer and its treatments can take their toll on your usual healthy relationship with food. It is particularly important during these times that you receive nutritious foods to replenish and nourish you. Ayurveda considers four foods to have particular rejuvenating value: milk, almonds, honey, and clarified butter. Some people do not tolerate milk due to a deficiency in lactase, the enzyme that digests milk sugar. However, our experience at the Chopra Center suggests that many people who consider themselves intolerant of milk can enjoy and benefit from this nutritious food if it is taken heated with spices such as ginger, cinnamon, and cardamom. If you are certain that you lack the enzyme to metabolize lactose, you can try milk that has lactase added or a milk substitute made from rice or soy. Support dairies that treat their cows compassionately and do not use hormones.

Ayurveda recommends eating a handful of almonds a day, which are an excellent source of protein, carbohydrates, and fiber. A delicious and nutritious shake can be made by combining three tablespoons of almond butter, one cup of milk, one tablespoon of honey, and one teaspoon of clarified butter in a blender. When you are having trouble forcing down solid food, drinking this nutritious shake will ensure that you are receiving some nourishment until your appetite returns.

Another nutritious and easy-to-digest dish recommended by Ayurveda is *kitchari*. Kitchari is a simple stew of rice and split mung beans prepared in about equal proportions. One-half cup of each slowly cooked in three cups of water makes a thin soup that can provide nourishment when no other food seems palatable. Add a little clarified butter, salt, and mild spices such as cumin, coriander, and fennel, and you will be surprisingly satiated. Stir in some chopped vegetables like carrots, green peppers, and tomatoes, and this simple meal will be rich in vitamins, minerals, and protein. Kitchari is an excellent food on days when you are undergoing chemotherapy and your digestion feels very delicate.

Let's summarize the important nutritional principles up to this point:

~ Follow a varied diet, rich in whole grains, fresh vegetables, and fruits.
~ Reduce your intake of animal protein and fat.
~ Ensure that you are receiving adequate essential amino acids through proper combinations of beans, grains, and vegetables.
~ Have all six tastes—sweet, sour, salty, pungent, bitter, astringent—at every meal.
~ If you are having symptoms of an excess in one of the three mind-body principles—wind, fire, or earth—favor the appropriate foods to create balance.
~ If your appetite or digestion is weak, use more bitter and pungent foods, herbs, and spices to enhance your digestive power.

~ If you are having symptoms of accumulated toxicity, follow a purifying diet.
~ If you are feeling debilitated, consume more replenishing foods.

Conscious Eating

As mentioned earlier in this chapter, our ability to digest food is as important as the quality of the food we eat. If our digestive power is inefficient, we are unable to fully benefit from even healthy, nutritious food. According to Ayurveda, how we prepare and consume food is as essential to its nourishing influence as its carbohydrate, protein, vitamin, and mineral composition.

There are some basic principles to follow regarding the preparation and eating of a meal. Paying attention to these simple principles can help you extract the highest levels of nourishment from everything you eat.

1. Eat your meals in a pleasant and comfortable environment. If your attention is distracted by chaotic surroundings, you digest the chaos along with your food. Don't engage in an argument or watch violent television shows or movies while eating. Love and appreciation are the best spices to use with every dish.

2. Don't eat when you are upset. A piece of cheesecake may seem the perfect choice right after a major argument with your mother, but your efforts to soothe your emotional upset with food will probably backfire. The powerful emotional chemicals released when you are experiencing emotional turmoil do not contribute to optimal digestion. Learn to process your feelings directly and wait until you feel less reactive before deciding to eat. Then, listen to your appetite and use food to fill your metabolic, not your emotional, needs.

3. Eat when you feel hungry. Your appetite is your best friend when it comes to nutrition. If you think of your appetite as a fuel gauge with zero being empty and ten being full, wait until you are at a level two or three before eating and then stop when you are at a six or seven. This means eating when you are hungry and stopping when you are comfortably full.

When facing cancer and while receiving treatment therapies, your appetite may be suppressed. During these times, try using fresh ginger or an appetite-enhancing apéritif before meals. Drink plenty of warm water and eat nutritiously whenever you feel hungry. Check in regularly with your bodily sensations and always eat with awareness.

4. Sip warm water with your meals. This helps the digestive process work efficiently. Reduce ice-cold foods and drinks, particularly when your digestion feels delicate. Our digestive enzymes are designed to work most efficiently at body temperature.

5. Eat freshly cooked meals. I've talked about Ayurveda's concept of life force, or *prana*, which is greater than the sum of the biochemicals that can be measured. The life force is greatest in meals prepared with fresh ingredients. Your body, mind, and soul will appreciate the time spent shopping for and preparing a luscious meal with fresh and attractive ingredients. The delicious smells and pleasing display of a freshly prepared meal stimulate the appetite and the secretion of digestive enzymes even before food is placed in the mouth. If you have to choose, I'd rather you spend time shopping for and cooking nourishing food than reading about the latest discovered benefits of a vitamin.

6. Reduce raw foods. Raw vegetables are richest in essential nutrients, and many dietary plans have emphasized their potential nutritional value. Unfortunately, our digestive power is often weakened when we are facing an illness. If we cannot readily assimilate the vitamins and minerals contained within raw foods, they are of little value to us. Steamed, baked, and lightly sautéed vegetables lose a little of their delicate nutrients, but appropriate cooking begins the digestive process, allowing us to extract greater nourishment from our food. Freshly prepared vegetable juices retain their nutrient content and are easier to assimilate than raw vegetables.

7. Sit quietly for a few minutes after your meal. Eating allows us to recreate ourselves. It is the process that enables us to take in the raw energy and information of the universe and transform it into the intelligence of our body. Savor the moments after a meal to appreciate the sacred act that is occurring.

Mindfulness Eating

Eating a meal with full awareness can be a powerful, enlightening, and healing experience. I recommend that you try this exercise and practice it at least once a week. Even though we have all been eating since the day we were born, most people who try this exercise learn something new about food.

~ Have the intention to eat a meal in silence: Begin the silence as you place your food on your plate. Become conscious of every intention and action. Notice the impulse that arises in your mind as you take a serving of each food. Notice the sounds, sensations, sights, and smells. Witness the motion of raising your utensil and consciously place a morsel in your mouth. Close your eyes and experience the flavors on your tongue. Become aware of the tastes and textures. Feel the sensations as you move the bolus of food to the back of your tongue and swallow it. See if you can trace the food as it moves down your esophagus into your stomach. Pause after each swallow and assess your level of satiety.

~ Continue eating each helping with your full awareness. Pace yourself so that you stay present with your meal. Monitor your level of fullness, and stop eating when you feel satisfied. Spend a few more minutes sitting quietly with your eyes closed, feeling the sensations in your mouth, throat, and stomach.

Many people notice that this exercise enlivens their taste sensations, reporting that the meal seems more vibrant with life energy. If someone is accustomed to overeating, they usually discover that they are satisfied earlier than they would have normally anticipated. If you eat your food consciously, it becomes nearly impossible to allow something unhealthy into your mouth. It seems that we are capable of consuming nutritionally empty substances only when we are distracted while eating by television, conversation, or work activities. If we cultivate the habit of eating consciously, we will enhance our enjoyment of meals and be more likely to eat healthy, nutritious foods.

Assessing Nutritional Programs

A vast array of dietary programs have been suggested for people facing cancer. Many of them are based upon providing foods that are believed to have cancer-fighting properties and encouraging the elimination of unwanted waste material. A garlic diet recommended by Hippocrates about 400 B.C. might have provided some benefit, considering that allicin, the active metabolite of garlic, induces mild anticancer activity. A diet consisting of grapes was popular in the 1500s in an effort to encourage elimination of toxic substances from the body, and we have recently learned that grapes are rich in certain cancer-fighting phytochemicals.[8]

The macrobiotic diet, introduced into the United States from Japan in the sixties, favors brown rice and cereal grains while avoiding animal products, including milk. A research group from Tulane Medical Center followed people with pancreatic and prostate cancer on a macrobiotic program and reported they had substantially better outcomes than would have been expected based upon the severity of their illnesses.[9] Although nutritionists have expressed concern about vitamin and mineral deficiencies in advanced stages of a macrobiotic diet, the Tulane group demonstrated that a nutritional plan consisting of whole grains, vegetables, beans, and soy products could meet the guidelines of both the National Research Council and the macrobiotic program. It has been suggested that a nutritionally deficient diet could be theoretically helpful to cancer patients by "starving" the malignant cells, but there is little evidence supporting this idea. In my experience a moderate macrobiotic dietary plan can be helpful in people who feel toxic and congested, but I would not encourage people who are debilitated to undergo intense nutritional restriction at a time when their bodies clearly need nourishment.

In 1958 Dr. Max Gerson, a German physician, published a book promoting his dietary plan for cancer, which favored fresh fruits and vegetables, whole grain breads, and mild cheeses.[10] Although components of the Gerson diet, such as liver injections and coffee enemas, are difficult to justify scientifically, the general principles of the diet were not that different from those of the American Cancer Society's current recommendations.

The more radical Kelly program, popular during the eighties, extended the approaches of the Gerson program to include pancreatic enzymes. Dr. William D. Kelly, a dentist, developed the theory that cancer resulted from the body's inability to digest protein, which could be remedied by taking enzyme supplements along with a restrictive diet. Unfortunately, there was little scientific support for the theory or any real evidence that supplemental enzymes were delivered to the cancer cells. I was a medical resident at University Hospital in San Diego when a Tijuana clinic based upon his principles was attracting Americans desperate for a simple answer to their illness. On a regular basis people with cancer were rushed across the border from Mexico to California for emergency treatment at our hospital. I would ask my somewhat reluctant patients why they were traveling thousands of miles to receive an unproved therapy that consisted primarily of a healthier diet. Most people expressed the sentiment that they had not rejected Western medicine so much as it had rejected them. They had been given little hope from their medical doctors and were seeking recognition of, and ways to mobilize, their body's own healing force. Even in the late seventies, people with cancer were looking for integrated approaches that used everything possible to improve their quality of life. Since Western medicine was locked in its material paradigm, many people sought out programs that offered some possibility for improving quality, if not quantity, of life. Fortunately, I believe we are starting to see a new openness to embracing body, mind, and spirit in the treatment of cancer.

I am certain that well-meaning people will continue to introduce new nutritional programs with claims to treat or cure cancer. It becomes very tempting to try such approaches, even if the basic theories or recommendations seem questionable or extreme. My suggestion is to use both your mind and your body to evaluate any new claim. Ask yourself if the basic approach makes sense to you. Does the dietary plan seem fairly natural and easy to follow? Is it balanced? Will you feel joy while following the program? If you decide to go on a new plan, listen to your body and hear whether the message is one of comfort and appreciation or strain and deprivation. Seek input from your health care providers and members of your cancer support network. If you honor the intelligence of both your mind and body, you will make appropriate decisions for your health.

Stop Driving Yourself Crazy

It is natural when people become ill to consider how diet is contributing to their problem. I hope it is obvious from this chapter that I firmly believe in the healing power of food. However, I do not believe in making eating so cumbersome that you fail to find any pleasure from the simple and elegant transformational process that is fundamental to life. Each day I see people who have been emphatically told by well-meaning nutritional advisors to avoid all dairy, sugars, salt, nightshade vegetables, acidic fruits, and wheat products. Their life is so restricted by these recommendations that they derive no enjoyment from eating.

If these restrictions result in tangible benefits, I am in full support of them. However, more often than not when I ask people if they have noticed positive effects from these austerities, I hear that they have developed intense cravings for these foods and feel worse than before. In appropriate settings it can be desirable to reduce heavier or sour foods, but it is rare that highly restricted diets can be sustained for long. My message regarding food is to trust your inner intelligence and seek out balance. If you find yourself straining to maintain a nutritional program, the stress of the diet is more than likely outweighing the benefits it is supposed to provide. Remember that eating is a sacred ritual, capable of providing nourishment to body, mind, and soul.

Listening to Our Bodies

In Ayurveda the body is called *anna maya kosha*, which means the layer of life composed of food. The biological intelligence carried in our genes directs the ingested raw material of the environment into the weaving of tissues we call our body. Ultimately, our body is made up of food wrapped around DNA. Just as weak lumber results in an unsound building, weak nutrition leads to an infirm body. To support healing, our diet must be balanced, nourishing, and digestible. It does not have to be complicated. I don't believe that Mother Nature expects us to have a degree in nutritional science to be able to nourish ourselves.

How much can we expect from nutrition when we are facing cancer? I think it's important to remember that food provides the building blocks for healing, but the patterns of intelligence that organize food into healthy tissues reside at a deeper level of our being. Food is the essence of our physical body, but it is not the essence of our being. To create an environment for healing, we need to establish the conditions for intelligence to flow effortlessly through the continuum of body, mind, and spirit. This means using every available option to create the possibility of wholeness and balance. To me, this includes the best of medical interventions along with optimal nutritional support and other holistic approaches that enliven our inner healer. Food alone cannot do everything, but it can begin the process of creating a healing milieu. Hippocrates said, "Let food be our medicine and medicine be our food," and like any remedy, the better prepared we are to benefit from the treatment, the more effective it will be.

Commitment to Wholeness

Our bodies are the end products of our experiences and interpretations. To change our bodies, we need to change our experiences. Make a commitment to change your life in the direction of greater love and caring for yourself and those close to you.

1. I consciously choose to eat foods that are nourishing, including more fresh fruits, vegetables, and whole grains and less animal fat. I will ensure that all six tastes are represented at every meal, while favoring those flavors that are balancing to my mind-body physiology.

2. I will pay attention to the way that I prepare and consume my meals, focusing on creating a nurturing environment that supports the celebration of eating.

3. I will eat at least one meal per week in silence, paying full attention to the smells, flavors, and visual presentation of my food and listening carefully to the signals my body is sending.

CHAPTER 4

Heroic Biochemicals

The Miracle and Mythology of Vitamins,
Minerals, and Other Healing Substances

What you eat is not the goal. What you are is the goal.—OSHO

Ellen survived her mastectomy and was tolerating her tamoxifen. She wanted to do everything possible to improve her chances for a healthy life, so she began studying nutritional approaches to cancer. She learned about free radicals and antioxidants and how some vitamins were helpful but might be harmful if taken in excess. She studied trace minerals and essential amino acids. She learned that sharks didn't get cancer and that drinking the juice of wheat grass could clear away her toxins. She heard that coffee was bad to drink but good for enemas, and that the reverse was true for tea. One source advised eating only raw vegetables and another advised eating only cooked ones. Trying to assimilate this information, she became increasingly frustrated. She learned that stress weakened her immune system and was beginning to wonder if all this nutritional advice designed to keep her healthy was actually making her sick.

Many years ago a friend of mine described the universe as an artichoke. He wasn't aware that his analogy was similar to the Vedic symbol of the universe—the lotus flower—representing the layers of life that unfold as we grow in awareness. An amazing aspect of having a human nervous system is that when we explore a subject more deeply we often discover a new realm of existence. This is true whether we are looking at a drop of pond water under a microscope, delving into the subatomic layers of matter, or investigating the health-enhancing effects of food. Most scientists are convinced that various diets can either lead to disease or promote well being. Now we are in a new phase, exploring *how* foods improve health. Nature seems willing to share her mysteries with us if we ask the right questions.

As we discovered in the last chapter, a diet rich in whole grains, vegetables, and fruits and low in animal fat provides a nutritional environment that is unfriendly to cancer. Although this may come as no surprise to those who intuitively recognize the value of a primarily vegetarian diet, fascinating new knowledge is emerging to explain how natural components of food enhance health. Looking into the artichoke at a deeper level reveals the wondrous intelligence inherent in nature's garden. I hope that sharing this information will help you avoid the confusion and frustration that Ellen and many other people facing cancer have experienced.

Vital Vitamins and Magnificent Minerals

Living on earth means living in a sea of oxygen. Every animal that has existed on our watery planet has required molecules of this gas to perform the basic metabolic functions necessary to sustain life. Comprising about 20 percent of our atmosphere at sea level, oxygen becomes an increasingly scarce commodity at rising altitudes, as most coastal dwellers quickly learn during their first few days in the Rocky Mountains. As children we used to see how long we could hold our breath, and we grasped firsthand that even though air is invisible, we could not go long without it.

We all understand the consequences of insufficient oxygen, but it is only fairly recently that we have begun to understand the dark side to our dependence on this essential gas. In almost every biochemical reaction that involves oxygen, we generate energetic molecules that have a brief but exciting life. Known as *free radicals*, these are not the vestiges of an underground antiwar movement, but rather, highly reactive chemicals with a strong need to unite with whatever is near and available. If not quickly neutralized, they assault the nearest protein, fat, carbohydrate, or gene, damaging its structure and altering its function. These highly reactive creatures are powerful, indiscriminate, and capable of wreaking havoc on our essential molecules.

In addition to normal biological reactions, free radicals are generated by our exposure to toxins. Smoking, air pollution, alcohol, radiation, trauma, infections, and burns all predispose us to create more free radicals, which translate insult into injury. These short-lived but dangerous gremlins take a variety of forms, but all have the potential to be destructive.

Free Radical Rascals

Superoxide radicals
Hydrogen peroxide
Singlet oxygen
Hypochlorous acid
Nitric oxide
Hydroxyl radicals

Fortunately, we have evolved a sophisticated and usually effective system to neutralize these troublesome by-products of living chemistry. Our antioxidant defense system consists of multiple levels of protection, including enzymes, vitamins, and trace metals. This brigade is essential to life, for we are under constant bombardment from free radicals. When our capacity to cancel out these damaging hooligans is unable to keep up with their production, we experience "oxidative stress." The damage to tissues that occurs as a result of the balance being tipped in favor of free radicals is linked to many common health problems, including rheumatoid arthritis, diseases of our blood vessels, and cancer. It has been estimated that our DNA is damaged by free radicals ten thousand times per day![1] With this high potential for genetic alteration, it's a testament to our remarkable repair systems that we are able to avoid cancer to the extent that we do. Anything we can offer our antioxidant troops to improve their defense capabilities benefits our health. And fortunately, there is growing evidence that foods we've already learned are good for us seem to be richest in antioxidant substances.

Vitamin C (Ascorbic Acid)

Vitamin C as a treatment for cancer became the cause of Nobel Prize winner Linus Pauling in the 1970s and '80s. With the discovery that most patients with cancer have lower-than-normal vitamin C levels in their blood, Pauling undertook a campaign to promote high doses of vitamin C for every cancer patient. Unfortunately, formal studies did not show a definite benefit in colon cancer, and enthusiasm for further research waned.[2] It is clear that vitamin C is a potent antioxidant with the ability to detoxify nitrates and nitrites, widely used food preservatives associated with cancer of the stomach. Vitamin C also seems to protect us from skin and lung cancer.[3]

Our richest sources of vitamin C are citrus fruits, tomatoes, berries, green peppers, potatoes, and leafy green vegetables. Sixty to one hundred milligrams per day are the Recommended Daily Allowances, although doses of up to twelve grams per day are suggested by megavitamin champions. If we choose to consume higher than the recommended allowances, our ability to absorb vitamin C falters. At an intake of two grams per day, we're able to absorb only one; if we go for the twelve grams suggested by megadose advocates, more than ten grams exit our body in the next bowel movement.

Vitamin C may have direct effects on our immunity, protecting our immune cells when they are actively trying to corral renegade cancer cells or infectious invaders. Although many people reach for vitamin C at the first sign of our most prevalent immune challenge—the common cold—scientific studies on its impact have been mixed.[4, 5]

What's my recommendation? Taking everything into consideration, I encourage my patients with cancer to take one gram of vitamin C per day in divided doses while they are undergoing cancer treatment and for three months afterward. In this range I feel confident they are receiving vitamin C's potential benefits with minimal risk of side effects.

Vitamin E

Eight closely related chemicals fall under the term *vitamin E*. The most powerful of these is alpha-tocopherol, which is found in vegetable oils, eggs, and whole grains. Vitamin E is a potent antioxidant that has been studied in cancer for over fifty years, with many but not all reports suggesting its benefit in the prevention and treatment of cancer.

A recent report showed that supplementation with 300 IU (200 milligrams) per day of vitamin E improved immune function in generally healthy elderly subjects.[6] This immune enhancement could also benefit people facing cancer. Studies in animals have shown that vitamin E may reduce the side effects of radiation and chemotherapy treatments. It may also work directly to slow the growth of tumors in a very interesting way. In chapter 1, I discussed how cancer cells seem to become deaf to the growth-controlling messages to which normal cells listen and respond.

Vitamin E seems to improve the ability of cancer cells to hear these messages of control.[7] As more research into this area unfolds, new approaches to cancer may be discovered.

Considering the possible benefits and minimal risk, I recommend daily supplementation with vitamin E at a dosage of three hundred international units (IU) during treatments and for a few months afterward. Although this is twenty times the Recommended Daily Allowance, doses of up to three thousand IU per day have been safely tolerated. Due to its potential protective effect during radiation and chemotherapy treatment, I would be certain to ensure adequate intake of vitamin E while you are receiving your treatments. If you are undergoing a course of radiation, massage your skin with olive or sunflower oil to which you've added vitamin E to provide an extra level of protection.

Vitamin A and the Carotenoids

Many studies over the years have shown that people with many different malignancies have lower vitamin A levels than people without cancer. Carotenoids are natural chemicals that can be converted into vitamin A, but we now know that these substances, present in many yellow, orange, and leafy green vegetables, have cancer-fighting potential of their own. The most common carotenoid in our diet is beta-carotene, found in high concentrations in carrots, cantaloupe, spinach, and broccoli. Beta-carotene and, to a lesser extent, vitamin A are effective free radical scavengers, but they also have other anticancer effects.[8] Like vitamin E, derivatives of vitamin A influence the way tumor cells respond to growth-regulating messenger molecules. Beta-carotene also seems to have the direct effect of waking up our immune cells.

Vitamin A in excessively high dosages can cause harm to our liver and nervous system, but we seem to safely tolerate beta-carotene, except for a reversible yellowing of the skin when it is taken in high doses. I recommend 25,000 IU of beta-carotene while you are receiving your cancer treatments. This dose will ensure that you are receiving adequate amounts of beta-carotene and vitamin A without approaching levels that have been associated with side effects or toxicity.

Although some oncologists have questioned whether antioxidant vitamins may interfere with the efficacy of radiation or chemotherapy, I am aware of no studies to date that support this concern. On the contrary, there have been several reports suggesting improved outcomes in people

Antioxidant Vitamin	Recommended Daily Allowance (RDA)	Recommended Dose during Treatment
Vitamin C	60 milligrams	1 gram
Vitamin E	15 IU	300 IU
Beta-carotene	None established	15 milligrams (25,000 IU)
Vitamin A	5000 IU	Derived from beta-carotene

receiving antioxidants while undergoing cancer treatments.[9–11] If your cancer doctors do not approve your use of antioxidants, I encourage you to follow their advice; but ask them for scientific support of their position. With careful attention to a balanced diet, we can receive ample essential nutrients, but when facing cancer, a person's weak appetite may make adequate intake challenging. Therefore, I suggest discussing the following recommendations on the use of supplemental antioxidant vitamins with your physician.

Winning Metals

A number of trace minerals are essential to ensure that our antioxidant enzymes work properly. Manganese, copper, zinc, and selenium are currently considered to be important in detoxifying free radicals and enhancing immune function.[12] Manganese and copper are abundant in leafy green vegetables, whole grains, legumes, and nuts. Zinc is present in whole grains and cereal, but the richest sources are of animal origin—milk, eggs, and meat.

Selenium has been receiving a lot of attention these days as an important antioxidant player. Studies have shown that geographical areas with high levels of selenium in the soil have lower rates of many cancers, including colon, lung, pancreatic, breast, and prostate.[13] A study from China showed that selenium had a protective effect in stomach and esophageal cancer.[14] In addition to its role in neutralizing free radicals, this essential mineral also stimulates our immune system. If the soil is rich in selenium, grains, beans, and vegetables are good sources. It is more concentrated in animal products such as seafood and organ meats.

The problem with trying to micromanage the intake of our mineral kingdom friends is that they tend to interact and compete with each other. A diet too high in zinc raises the risk of a copper deficiency. Manganese competes with many other minerals, including calcium, copper, iron, and zinc, for uptake into our digestive tract. Copper and zinc are slightly competitive with selenium.

So, what should we do regarding these necessary metals? Taking into account the available information, I recommend a well-balanced mineral supplement during the period of your cancer treatments. Particularly if your appetite is suppressed, supplementing with a multimineral formula is prudent. I do not recommend taking high doses of a single vitamin or mineral because of the close interrelations among the various nutrients. In our desire to maximize the potential benefit of one trace element, we may cause imbalances in another. A balanced formula like the one below is readily available from your pharmacy or health food store.

Mineral	Dose
Calcium	1 gram
Iron	18 milligrams
Magnesium	400 milligrams
Manganese	5 milligrams
Chromium	100 micrograms
Iodine	150 micrograms
Molybdenum	100 micrograms
Copper	2 milligrams
Zinc	15 milligrams
Selenium	100 micrograms

Does Nutrition Have to Be So Complicated?

It is easy to understand how anyone seeking a nutritional approach to health can become confused. I was recently in a health food store and overheard a conversation between the clerk in the vitamin section and a woman who was trying to solicit his advice on how much vitamin E, if any, she should be taking. He began his response by telling her of some recent studies that suggested vitamin E might protect against Alzheimer's disease in higher doses than that recommended for people with heart disease. If she wanted to take vitamin E for premenstrual syndrome, he advocated a lower dose. Although most people recommend alpha-tocopherol, he informed her that some people are now promoting gamma-tocotrienol as the most potent form, particularly if she wanted to lower her cholesterol level. By this point, the poor woman became frustrated and decided that the multiple vitamin she had at home would be more than adequate.

Our linear approach to health often fails to embrace the understanding that life is interrelated and contextual. A study may attempt to isolate the role of a single nutrient on health, but it is impossible to ignore the interweaving of the many facets of nutrition. This is why I believe that nature is the best source of healing wisdom. We know that a diet low in animal fat, high in whole grains, fruits, vegetables, and fiber protects us from cancer. At a biochemical level, we learn that these same foods are rich in vitamins and minerals and important in neutralizing toxic chemicals, enhancing our immune system, and possibly bringing cancer cells under control. We can obtain these necessary health-enhancing nutrients through a balanced wholesome diet, and the joy we feel in eating a delicious meal generates its own life-supporting influence.

My bottom line recommendation is to eat a diet rich in grains, legumes, vegetables, and fruits, ensuring that all six tastes are available. During your cancer treatments, when your appetite may be delicate, and for a few months afterwards, supplement your diet with a good balanced multivitamin that supplies the important antioxidant vitamins along with a good multimineral formula. Most important, enjoy the experience of eating, as it is a true celebration of life.

Fabulous Phytochemicals

I recently shopped for a sport coat at a department store. I was having difficulty making a decision because the coat I thought would best meet my needs was almost twice as expensive as my second choice. I finally decided to go for the more expensive one and with some misgiving brought my choice to the purchase counter. There the clerk delighted me with the news that my coat was on sale for 50 percent off! I made what I thought was the best choice and then received an unanticipated boon.

In a similar way, new information on the health-promoting natural chemicals in edible plants is showing us that we are getting a lot more healing energy from our vegetables and fruits than we ever imagined. *Phytochemicals* (*phyto* in Greek means plant) is the name applied to thousands of naturally occurring substances found in grains, beans, vegetables, and fruits. Phytochemicals contribute to the color and flavor of plants while providing them with resistance to viruses, fungi, and other plant adversaries. When we ingest a plant-rich diet, these phytochemicals provide us with health-enhancing benefits in many different ways.

One class of plant chemicals, *isothiocyanates*, is found in high concentrations in cruciferous vegetables, including Brussels sprouts, broccoli, cabbage, and cauliflower. These seem to inhibit enzymes that activate carcinogens and increase enzymes that neutralize toxic substances.[15] Another class of phytochemicals, *flavonoids*, are potent antioxidants and inhibit tumor development. They are abundant in citrus fruits, berries, carrots, and potatoes. Flavonoids seem to reduce the ability of cancer to spread and blunt the effect of hormones on cancer cells.[16] The flavonoid compound *silymarin*, found in artichokes, has been shown to protect animals from skin cancer. Strawberries, grapes, and walnuts contain *ellagic acid*, which neutralizes carcinogens and blocks their gene-damaging effect. In one study, laboratory rats fed a diet rich in ellagic acid had less than half the esophageal tumors of animals fed a regular diet.[17] As a final example, *capsaicin*, the chemical found in hot peppers, is an effective antioxidant and protects our DNA from cancer-causing damage. Several of the major phytochemical groups are described below.[18]

Phytochemical	Sources	Actions
Isothiocyanates	Broccoli, Brussels sprouts, cabbage, cauliflower, kale, turnips, watercress	Blocks carcinogens; inhibits tumor growth
Flavonoids	Citrus fruits, apples, beans, onions, broccoli	Antioxidants; blocks carcinogens, blocks cancer-stimulating hormones
Phenolic compounds	Vegetables, fresh fruits, berries, tea, broccoli, nuts	Antioxidants; inhibits tumor growth
Monoterpenes	Orange peel, cherries, garlic, sage, dill	Blocks carcinogens; inhibits growth-promoting proteins
Lignans	Whole grains, flaxseed, fruits, vegetables	Antioxidants; blocks cancer-stimulating hormones

Once again, scientific information on the healing power of food is both fascinating and intimidating. If we are facing cancer, should we focus on specific phytochemicals in an effort to influence our internal chemical environment? It probably won't be long before individual flavonoids, phenols, and lignans are for sale at our local health food store. However, I believe nature intended us to receive the healing energy of plants through the beautifully packaged fruits, vegetables, grains, herbs, and spices that grow in our planetary garden. I am repeatedly impressed with how the simple nutritional principles of Ayurveda remain relevant today:

~ Eat a variety of foods representing all the major tastes.
~ Favor freshly prepared vegetables, grains and legumes.
~ Prepare food so it is enticing and delicious.

If we follow these principles, we will ensure that our diet provides the best environment for health and healing. I am in full agreement with a recent position statement by the American Academy of Pediatrics that concluded, "Good food is better than good pills."[19]

Commitment to Wholeness

Our bodies are the end products of our experiences and interpretations. To change our bodies, we need to change our experiences. Make a commitment to change your life in the direction of greater love and caring for yourself and those close to you.

1. I will choose nourishing foods, with more fruits, vegetables, and whole grains and less animal fat. Ensuring all six tastes are represented gives me confidence that I will be receiving the essential vitamins, minerals, and phytochemicals.

2. While I am undergoing treatment for my illness, I will ensure that I am receiving plentiful health-enhancing nutrients. If I choose to use nutritional supplements, I will do so in a balanced and rational way.

3. I will not substitute dietary supplements for nutritionally rich foods. I will view vitamins, minerals, and other nutritional fortifiers as complementary to a healthy, balanced diet.

CHAPTER 5

The Wisdom of Herbs

Accessing Nature's Botanical Intelligence

And the earth brought forth grass and herb yielding seed . . . and God
saw that it was good.—GENESIS 1:12

Isabella and Ferdinand were having problems with their health.
The political world that consumed their lives was exacting a toll
on their well being. They were both experiencing a lot of stress
due to ongoing political conflicts. Isabella was having trouble
with her digestion and was barely sleeping at night. Ferdinand's
heartburn was acting up, and his gouty arthritis was flaring.

They heard that there were medicinal herbs from the Far East
that would alleviate their problems, but their physician was having difficulty locating a reliable source. Then an adventurous en-
trepreneur approached Isabella and Ferdinand, seeking financial
support for a project to access a steady supply of herbs and spices
from India. For both personal and economic reasons, they decided to fund the project. So, an explorer with the name Christo-
pher Columbus was given the backing of the royalty of Spain to
find a shortcut to the botanical riches of India.

Since before written history, human beings have been sampling their
environmental garden, seeking remedies for the inevitable health challenges of life. A good part of this process was through trial and error. A
nibble from a country mallow shrub resulted in a burst of sustained energy, while a tea made from valerian roots induced sleep. After a meal of
wild boar a dose of chamomile flowers relieved indigestion, and a few

leaves of senna resulted in a prompt and potent evacuation. One can hardly imagine what our ancestral herbalists must have thought after innocently consuming a bite of psilocybin mushroom or inhaling some jimsonweed tossed onto a fire. Herbs and spices have been an integral component of every healing tradition in the world and were of prime importance in the West until fairly recently. With the advent of modern pharmacology and our focus on disease-specific treatments, the role of natural medicines was relegated to second-class status. And yet, much of the richness of our modern pharmacopoeia comes from our botanical kingdom. At least 25 percent of drugs prescribed by medical doctors are derivatives of herbal medicines.[1] Aspirin and morphine for pain, atropine, quinidine, and digitalis for our heart, colchicine for gout, psyllium and castor oil for our gut, taxol and vincristine for cancer—these are just a few of the more than 150 modern medicines that have their roots in the herbal kingdom.

What happened to shift Western medicine so far away from the vast treasure house of natural healing substances? One of our first steps away from the supremacy of herbs was the discovery of potent antibiotics that could quickly and effectively eliminate life-threatening infections. When penicillin and sulfa drugs were discovered in the 1920s and '30s, we began believing that we could find a pharmaceutical agent for every disease. This has, of course, led to phenomenal advances in the treatment of illness. Our understanding of the mechanisms of disease has expanded at an unprecedented pace, and almost every week a new disorder is understood in genetic or molecular terms. Our modern therapeutic approach strives to isolate an active ingredient, enabling us to specifically interfere with a disease process to the extent that we understand it. It's a fundamental principle of modern medicine to use a single active chemical whenever possible, although with some infections and most cancers, a multiple chemical attack is the rule. Because almost every medicinal herb is composed of multiple chemicals, our Western scientific approach is flustered by nature's shotgun ways.

Traditional herbal medicine resists a linear approach, believing that nature has packaged herbs to maximize their benefit and minimize their toxicity. Dr. James Duke recently emphasized the complexity of herbal medicines in his discussion on bilberry for arthritis.[2] A close cousin of the blueberry, this plant contains nineteen phytochemicals that may help arthritis, including pain relievers, anti-inflammatories, and antioxidants. We could try to isolate the one most potent component, but we might then lose the synergy that the combination provides. In many cases, an ingredient that was thought to be inert turns out to be important in enhancing absorption or reducing toxicity of the active phytochemical. A good example of this is the widely used heart medicine digitalis. Derived from foxglove, this cardiac fortifier was known in ancient India, China, Egypt, and Rome. When the dried leaves of foxglove were the most common way to administer this herbal medicine, an early sign of toxicity was appetite loss, nausea, and vomiting. This was a warning to physicians to reduce the dosage before more serious side effects appeared. Today, the earliest expression of digitalis toxicity is often a potentially life-threatening heart rhythm disturbance. One explanation for this is that the most common form of digitalis now prescribed is a refined derivative called digoxin. This purified medicine does not have the other "inactive" components of the original plant that provide the digestive warning symptoms when the dosage is too high. We have extracted the intelligence, but discarded the wisdom, of the herb. Medical doctors now need to monitor the amount of digoxin in the blood, so we'll know if the patient is approaching a toxic range. Technology creates the need for greater technology.

I am not suggesting that we should toss out pharmaceuticals and replace them with herbs. The evolution of modern drugs has been a rational and evolutionary process. A physician wants to know that the medicine she is prescribing is of consistent purity and potency. This is very difficult to ensure with herbs. Plants from one area may have concentrations of healing constituents different from the same plant from another locale or when harvested in a different season. While in India recently, meeting with the head of a leading Ayurvedic herbal company, I was told they were cultivating rare Himalayan herbs in petri dishes, then raising them in greenhouses under ideal conditions. Shrubs seen rarely over a foot high in the mountains were growing into six-foot-high bushes in their greenhouses. This seemed at first like a real breakthrough in technology, but we began to wonder if the medicinal effect of an herb grown in a "cushy" greenhouse would be equivalent to one that had to struggle to survive in a harsh, austere environment. We are just beginning to develop the technology to answer these kinds of questions.

As should be apparent by now, I do not believe that the answers lie in an either/or approach. For many cancers, herbal medicine cannot approach the potential efficacy of modern chemotherapy agents. Therefore, we use the tool that is most appropriate for the task. However, there are many important benefits that herbs can offer to people facing cancer, including reducing the side effects of treatment, enhancing immune function, and improving the overall quality of life. The integration of modern and holistic approaches helps create the best environment for healing.

Rational Use of Herbs

Herbs and spices can be powerful healing tools when used appropriately. Before exploring the various ways herbal medicines can be therapeutic, I'd like to examine a few basic ideas about natural remedies.

1. Herbs are medicines. If an herb has a specific health influence, it does so on the basis of its biochemical effect even if we don't precisely understand the scientific mechanism. There is a rational explanation for an herb that improves digestion, enhances elimination, or stimulates immune function. We don't need to think of herbs as having mystical powers for us to honor and use them.

2. Not all herbs are powerful medicines. In every natural healing tradition, certain herbs are held in high esteem and others are considered minor. Nature does not always package medicines in a high-potency form. There may be validity to a traditional claim for an herb, and it's appropriate to critically evaluate the assertion. For example, it is commonly held that willow bark is an effective antiarthritis herb because of its content of salicylates. However, in order to get enough pain reliever equivalent to two aspirin, we'd have to consume over ten grams of powdered bark.[3] This might require more than half a gallon of willow bark tea!

3. Herbs can be toxic and have side effects. Just because something is natural doesn't mean it is completely harmless. Anyone who's had a brush with poison ivy understands this principle. Plants have evolved powerful chemicals to protect themselves from infections and predators. Some of these phytochemicals are beneficial, and some are potentially harmful.[4] We need to use herbs responsibly to maximize their benefit to us.

4. Most herbs are best used for a limited period of time. Although rejuvenating herbs may be used on a daily basis, most natural medicines should be taken over a defined treatment course. If the health problem resolves, the herb should be stopped. If the problem persists, another approach needs to be considered. For example, I do not advise people to

regularly take echinacea to stimulate their immunity, for it then seems to be less effective when they are facing an immune challenge. Food is taken daily; medicinal herbs are taken when needed.

5. The quality of an herb determines its effectiveness. Fresh herbs are generally more potent than dried ones, and every substance has a limited life expectancy. An appropriately chosen herb that has been sitting on the shelf for several years is unlikely to have the anticipated therapeutic benefit. Unfortunately, there is little standardization in this area, and it may be impossible to determine an herb's expiration date. Whenever possible, try using natural medicines within six to twelve months of their harvesting.

Herbs in Cancer Care

What help can herbs offer to people facing cancer? Several important chemotherapy drugs are derived from plants. The most recent one to receive attention is taxol, derived from the Pacific yew tree. Taxol has been used successfully in women with ovarian cancer, but like most cancer medicines it suppresses the bone marrow and causes nausea. Another cancer drug, etoposide, comes from the mayapple plant and is used to treat lung and testicular tumors. The periwinkle plant has given us vincristine and vinblastine, both used in the treatment of lymphomas. Many other plants, such as custard apple, Bauhinia, barberry, and Indian olibaum, have been shown to change the way cancer cells reproduce when grown in laboratory cultures, but we don't yet know how important these effects are in human beings.

General Immune
Enhancers (Adaptogens)

Although Jim had completed his treatment for testicular cancer four months ago, he continued to be frustrated by his lack of vitality. Despite sleeping nine hours at night, he routinely felt lethargic in the morning and inevitably needed to take a nap in the early afternoon. He had been meditating daily and was eating a balanced diet when I saw him in consultation. I recommended

General Immune Enhancers

English name	Ayurvedic/Chinese medicine name	Latin name	Dosage
Echinacea	—	*Echinacea augustifolia*	¼ to ½ gram twice per day
Astragalus	Yellow vetch	*Astragalus mongollicus*	½ gram twice per day
Winter cherry	Ashwagandha	*Withania somnifera*	½ gram twice per day

that he begin taking ginseng and ashwagandha as general fortifiers. Over the course of the next few weeks he noticed a gradual but steady improvement in his energy level. Although he began sleeping less, he felt that his endurance was better. He believed that these tonic herbs were nourishing him at a subtle but important level.

There are a number of herbs that can enhance our immune function and may prove valuable for people facing cancer. These herbal medicines are also sometimes known as adaptogens, biological response modifiers, or simply tonics. In Ayurveda, they are called *rejuvenatives*, or *rasayanas* in Sanskrit. The most popular immune-enhancing Western herb is echinacea. Used by many Native American tribes, several studies have demonstrated that it can stimulate immune cells to engulf invading organisms.[5] It is most commonly used to prevent and treat viral infections. While undergoing cancer treatments that weaken your natural immunity, keep some echinacea close at hand to be used at the first sign of infection.

Astragalus root, widely used in traditional Chinese medicine, is another general resistance enhancer. It seems to have widespread effects on immune function, including stimulating the maturation of immune cells, increasing the production of interferon, and intensifying the potency of macrophages.[6] This herbal medicine can be safely used to ward off colds and influenza.

The Ayurvedic herb ashwagandha is known in English as winter cherry. It has a long history in India as an enhancer of immunity, with recent studies lending credibility to these ancient claims. Ashwagandha con tains many unique phytochemicals, some of which activate macrophages and their enzymes. Animal studies have shown that some of the many chemicals contained in this complex herb have antitumor activity.[7] It is now readily available in the United States from a number of herbal sources. Ashwagandha is considered a rejuvenative in Ayurveda that can be taken on a sustained basis to improve overall well being.

Digestive Aids

A strong appetite, balanced digestion, and regular elimination are essential aspects of good health and are of particular importance in people facing illness. The emotional stress of cancer, the disease itself, and the treatments can all negatively impact the digestive process. Simple nutritional herbal supplements can help to reestablish balance in the gastrointestinal system and improve overall well being.

There are two types of herbs to improve appetite and digestion—those with bitter and those with pungent tastes. Bitter tonics have been used for thousands of years in China and India and more recently in the West. The bitter taste makes us salivate, stimulates stomach acid secretion, and induces our stomach to empty. All these effects can be used to strengthen a weak appetite and digestion. The classical bitter tonic is gentian, derived from the roots and underground stems of several closely related plants. It is also the basis for some alcoholic "bitters" used to stimulate the appetite before a meal. Other useful bitter herbs that can improve appetite and digestion include quinine, goldenseal, and aloe vera. A bitter Ayurvedic herb, extolled in India and now readily available in the West, is neem (Azadiracta indica). In addition to its use as a digestive stimulant, neem is traditionally used to treat bacterial, viral, and fungal infections.

Pungent herbs are also beneficial digestive aids. Fresh gingerroot taken before a meal stimulates the appetite and improves digestive power. The fresh juice combined with lemon juice and honey makes a delicious natural apéritif. In Ayurveda, dried ginger is combined with equal parts black pepper and long pepper to create a formula known as *trikatu*, meaning "three pungents." Taken a half hour prior to a meal, it is designed for people with a weak appetite and for those with weak digestion.

Aromatic pungent herbs can also help to reduce nausea. Studies on ginger showed it to be effective for morning sickness in pregnancy and in reducing motion sickness.[8] I recommend its liberal usage while people

Reducing Nausea, Improving Digestion

English name	Ayurvedic name	Latin name	Dosage
Bitter herbs			
Gentian	Kirata	*Gentiana species*	$1/4$ to $1/2$ gram as needed
Goldenseal	—	*Hydrastis canadensis*	$1/4$ gram twice per day
Aloe	Kumari	*Aloe vera*	$1/2$ ounce juice twice per day
Neem	Nimba	*Azadiracta indica*	$1/4$ to $1/2$ gram twice per day
Pungent herbs			
Ginger	Andraka	*Zingiber officinale*	$1/4$ tsp. grated root before meals
Cloves	Lavanga	*Caryophyllus aromaticus*	1 bud as needed for nausea
Cinnamon	Twak	*Cinnamomum zeylanicum*	Small piece of bark as needed
Mint	Phudina	*Mentha species*	1 tbsp. per cup of water infusion

are undergoing chemotherapy treatments in the form of a tea using one-half teaspoon of grated gingerroot per cup of hot water. Other aromatic herbs that can help reduce nausea are cloves, cinnamon, and peppermint. Try sucking on a whole clove or a natural cinnamon stick when your stomach is queasy, or sipping a cup of peppermint tea. When your upper digestive tract is sluggish, the essential oils in these herbs help dispel heaviness, congestion, and mucus. Fortunately, very powerful and effective antivomiting medications are now available when potent chemotherapy drugs that cause nausea are required.

Balancing Elimination

Carl was uncomfortable. He was requiring regular doses of narcotic medication to treat the pain in his spine and had not had a bowel movement for five days. He was asking to increase his pain medicine, but when I learned of his constipation, I suggested we first try to get his digestive tract moving. Using a combination of stool softeners, psyllium, and a small dose of senna, he was finally able to evacuate. His pain immediately lessened, and he was actually able to reduce his medication. With plenty of fluids, a high-fiber diet, and triphala, his bowels became more regular and he was much more comfortable.

Constipation is a common problem that can become worse when facing a serious illness. Elimination problems, which are common in people dealing with cancer, add additional, and usually unnecessary, suffering. Attending to this problem can often improve both digestive health and general well being. The stress of cancer and the many medications used to treat it frequently cause the bowels to be sluggish. Although I learned in medical school that a daily bowel movement is not a requirement for good health, I have repeatedly seen people's well being improve when they are eliminating once a day. Regular movements are essential to ensure that wastes and toxins are removed from the body.

There are many herbal remedies available to improve bowel function, but the most important approach is to follow a diet high in natural fiber. Plenty of fresh fruits, vegetables, and whole grains are the keys to keeping our digestive tract moving. If your bowels are becoming sluggish, the first step is to increase your intake of fiber. Bran is one of the richest sources, followed by fruits, vegetables, and legumes. Be sure to drink plenty of water while taking prunes or dried fruit to increase the bulk in your intestines. Psyllium seeds can provide a reliable fiber source but must be taken with lots of fluids. Flaxseed is another excellent herbal source that can be used as a tea before bedtime. Increasing your intake of natural oils such as sesame, almond, and olive will help soften the stool.

If these simpler measures are unsuccessful, you may need to use an herb that has a laxative effect. These products work by increasing fluid in the bowel and stimulating the nerves to the colon, and there are many to choose from. Cascara, rhubarb, aloe, and senna are the most widely used medicinal plants. Castor oil works similarly but has a stronger and faster cathartic effect. Cascara sagrada is probably the gentlest of these plants, although teas made from senna are widely available. It's a general principle that these stimulant laxatives should not be used on a regular basis as they can create cramping and electrolyte imbalances, but they can be very

Elimination Enhancers

English name	Ayurvedic name	Latin name	Dosage
Psyllium	Snigdhajira	*Plantago psyllium*	1 tsp. seeds in 1 cup water
Flaxseed	Uma	*Linum usitatissimum*	1 tsp. seeds in 1 cup water
Senna	Markandika	*Cassia acutifolia*	$\frac{1}{2}$ to 1 gram dried leaves in 1 cup water
Cascara	—	*Cascara sagrada*	$\frac{1}{2}$ to 1 gram dried bark in 1 cup water

useful to get the digestive tract moving until gentler dietary changes can take effect.

Diarrhea

During cancer therapy, it is not uncommon to go through a period of diarrhea. Chemotherapy medicines work on cells that are rapidly multiplying, which includes those that line our digestive tract. The cells in our intestines may be temporarily injured by the medications, resulting in diarrhea. Herbs with the astringent taste, reflecting a high content of tannins, are effective natural approaches to slow down digestive function. Tannins bind to injured cells, acting like a chemical Band-Aid. However, tannin-rich herbs should be used sparingly and for a limited time, for they can be toxic if used excessively. Also, we may not want to stop loose stools completely, for diarrhea may be our body's attempt to detoxify. We can lose a lot of water quickly through loose stools, so it's always important to replenish fluids that are lost with a balanced electrolyte solution. If the problem does not resolve promptly, contact your physician so the specific cause can be determined and appropriate treatment provided.

Fenugreek and pomegranate are traditional Ayurvedic remedies that are readily available in the West. Dried raspberry, blueberry, and blackberry leaves are rich in tannins and are well-known antidiarrhea remedies in Western herbology. A common over-the-counter remedy for simple diarrhea is the combination of the fine clay, kaolin, with pectin, derived from vegetable and fruit fiber. Most widely recognized as Kaopectate,

Slowing Things Down

English name	Ayurvedic name	Latin name	Dosage
Fenugreek	Methi	*Trigonella foenumgraeceum*	1/4 to 1/2 gram two to four times per day
Pomegranate	Dadima	*Punica granatum*	Four ounces of fresh juice four times per day
Raspberry leaves	—	*Rubus species*	1 tbsp. per cup of water infusion
—	Triphala	*Emblica officinalis, Terminalia chebula, Terminalia bellerica*	Two tablets containing 1/3 gram each before bedtime

this product is thought to work by absorbing extra fluid and protecting the inner lining of the intestines.

The most effective antidiarrhea agents are derived from opium, which comes from the juice of the poppy flower. Known for thousands of years, we use many opium-derived medicines for pain relief, and now understand that their power comes from mimicking our brain's natural pain relievers. Most opiates that slow the bowels require a prescription from your doctor, but loperamide, a synthetic opiate, can be purchased over the counter. Again, before using any medicine, be certain to communicate with your health care provider.

Within Ayurvedic herbology a combination formula of three dried fruits is considered to be a general bowel tonic. Known in Sanskrit as *triphala* (tri = three, phala = fruit), it combines amalaki (*Emblica officinalis*), haritaki (*Terminalia chebula*), and bibhitaki (*Terminalia bellerica*). These fruits are reported to improve elimination function whether a person's bowels are too loose or too hard. This combination is now widely available from a number of herbal companies and can be taken on a daily basis.

Cooling Inflamed Membranes

Donna noticed an irritation at the back of her tongue that persisted for several weeks. When it failed to resolve spontaneously, she saw her ear, nose, and throat specialist, who took a biopsy of the irritated site. The results returned positive for squamous cell carcinoma, and a course of radiation therapy was recommended. Her radiation therapist told her to expect inflammation of her mucous membranes and warned her there was a possibility she might need a feeding tube for a time. She came to see us at the Chopra Center, hoping there was some alternative to radiation therapy.

After reviewing her situation, I agreed that the radiation offered the best opportunity to eliminate the cancer, but thought that there might be some interventions that could reduce the side effects. I advised her to gargle several times daily with herbalized sesame oil and to swish her mouth with aloe vera juice before and after each treatment. She also received dietary advice to minimize sour foods during her treatment and to drink licorice tea. To everyone's pleasant surprise she easily sailed through her radiation treatments without any significant toxicity and was declared cancer-free six months later.

Would she have had as easy a course without the recommendations? Until we have well-designed scientific studies, we won't know the answer. I do know that she felt much more confident proceeding with the treatments, believing she was actively doing something to enhance her health.

During cancer therapy, the inner lining of the mouth can become inflamed and irritated from drugs and radiation. Known as mucositis, it can be very uncomfortable, make adequate nutrition difficult, and increase susceptibility to infections. Gargling with a soothing herbal mouthwash can provide symptomatic relief and may hasten healing. Most herbs used for inflamed mucous membranes are astringent in taste with a high tannin content. Western herbs used this way include sage, goldenseal, and raspberry leaf. Slippery elm, marshmallow, and Solomon's seal share a lubricating and cooling effect and can be used liberally. Licorice is moistening and has an anti-inflammatory effect. Neem is one of the most powerful cooling herbs in the Ayurvedic pharmacy and also helps to fight infections. The best way to use these soothing herbs is to make a strong infusion by adding a couple of tablespoons of the herb to one cup of boiling water and then letting it set until cool. Strain the herb and gargle with the liquid several times a day.

Membrane Soothers

English name	Ayurvedic name	Latin name	Dosage
Sage	—	*Salvia officinalis*	2 tbsp. dried leaves in 1 cup water infusion
Slippery elm	—	*Ulmus fulva*	2 tbsp. dried bark in 1 cup water infusion
Licorice	Yasti madhu	*Glycyrrhiza glabra*	2 tbsp. dried chopped roots in 1 cup water infusion
Neem	Nimba	*Azadiracta indica*	2 tbsp. dried leaves in 1 cup water infusion

Calming the Mind

Throughout this book I'll be discussing ways to bring your attention beyond the level of noise to a place of quietness and trust. In this tranquil state, our minds induce our brains to send the most healing influences to our body. Meditation, yoga, and visualizations are the most powerful means to access expanded awareness infused with inner silence. However, in the midst of the challenges of facing cancer, there may be times when it seems that our worries and anxieties have a life of their own. There are few experiences more distressing than feeling exhausted at night but unable to fall asleep because your mind is racing. In these situations, a natural herbal sedative can take the edge off mental agitation, enabling you to get some much-needed rest. Calming herbs are sometimes referred to in Western herbology as nervines.

The most widely known calming herb in the West, with over a thousand-year history of usage, is valerian. Although the precise mechanism of its action remains unknown, it has been shown to have measurable sedative properties in animals and humans.[9] Other commonly used Western nervines include skullcap, hops, passionflower, and chamomile.

Ayurveda has its own rich pharmacy of natural calming herbs. Indian valerian, known in Sanskrit as *jatamansi* (*Nardostachys jatamansi*), is a gentle, effective sedative that reduces restlessness and is helpful in insomnia. In addition to taking jatamansi internally, it can also be used as an herbal potpourri. An ounce of dried ground roots and underground stems is placed in a small silk pillow and the sachet is inhaled as you lie down to rest. Children particularly love this approach.

Brahmi and shankhapushpi are two other Ayurvedic herbs used to calm the mind. Many different herbs in India have received the name brahmi, referring to their influence on consciousness (brahm = seat of consciousness). Gotu kola *(Hydrocotyle asiatica)*, readily available in the West, is sometimes referred to as brahmi, but tends to have an alerting effect on the mind. The most widely used form of brahmi in India, *Bacopa monniera*, is available in the United States and has a demonstrable sedative effect.[10] Shankhapushpi *(Canscora decussata)* is another important Ayurvedic nervine that is also used to treat nerve and rheumatic pain. A combination formula of jatamansi, brahmi, and shankhapushpi makes a wonderful, gentle sleeping aid that does not cause drowsiness in the morning.

A very simple sleep-inducing aid is to prepare some hot milk with a pinch of nutmeg or cardamom. Although the amino acid L-tryptophan is no longer available as a sole supplement, milk is a rich source of this calming essential biochemical. It's been recently suggested that other chemicals in milk may generate endorphinlike activity, perhaps explaining why nursing babies always seem to be in bliss.[11]

These calming herbs can be very helpful in quieting mental turbulence. They are not, however, the equivalent of potent sleeping or anti-anxiety medications such as diazepam (Valium) or alprazolam (Xanax). If you have been requiring one of these psychoactive medications, do not abruptly discontinue it. Rather, with the approval of your doctor, add one of these gentle calming herbs and assess its influence on you. If after some time you feel you are ready to reduce or eliminate a prescribed medication, do so under the direct guidance of your physician. Although I often see people who notice some benefit from a natural approach and wish to quickly eliminate all medications, I do not believe this is safe or prudent. If you are gaining benefit from a natural remedy, its value should become increasingly obvious over time. Gradually weaning off a medication is the safest route and will avoid any rebound complications that may occur if a drug is stopped too quickly.

Ancient Medicines, Modern Times

In the honoring of herbs, I believe it's important not to expect more from these botanical gifts than they can deliver. In simpler times, we were not swimming in the chemical soup of a modern urban environment. At times, the chemically provoked diseases of our day may require more powerful pharmaceuticals than nature may spontaneously provide. Ayurveda addresses this issue by describing six stages of illness. The initial steps are reflective of early imbalance and can be more easily reversed through simple adjustments in diet, daily routine, and herbs. If the disease progresses to a more manifest state, subtler interventions have less of an effect, and more potent tools may be required.

Our botanical friends provide protection from the onslaught of cancer-causing agents that surround us and help create a favorable healing environment. For distressing symptoms that reflect disruption of our basic life functions such as eating, eliminating, and sleeping, herbs should be the first choice in an effort to establish balance. Drugs should be resorted to only if these natural healing substances do not provide relief. In my experience, herbal medicine is a valuable complement to, but not a substitute for, appropriate medical care. Whenever possible, use the subtlest approach that will provide benefit, and be open to all possibilities that can enhance your recovery.

Commitment to Wholeness

Our bodies are the end products of our experiences and interpretations. To change our bodies, we need to change our experiences. Make a commitment to change your life in the direction of greater love and caring for yourself and those close to you.

1. I will create my own herbal collection using nature's remedies as needed to help normalize my digestion, elimination, and sleeping patterns.

2. I will use herbs respectfully and appropriately. I will not expect more from them than they are capable of providing, and I will not underestimate their ability to help balance and nourish my mind and body.

3. I will stay open to using the best tool available for any health problem I may encounter, communicating candidly and honestly with my health care provider.

CHAPTER 6

Contending with Cancer

*Complementary Approaches for Coping
with Symptoms and Side Effects*

There is no coming to consciousness without pain.—CARL JUNG

Can I see another's woe,
And not be in sorrow too?
Can I see another's grief,
And not seek for kind relief?
—WILLIAM BLAKE

You don't need to be reminded that facing cancer is not a pleasure sport. The road to recovery from cancer is strewn with rocks and potholes, often taxing your navigational skills. Because of the many challenges cancer brings, I believe it's important to remain open to all possibilities that may improve your quality of life. As is the case with a pregnant woman in labor, facing a serious illness is no time for dogmatism. It's nice to think that we could get by without the need for any medical intervention, but this is seldom realistic or helpful. Similarly, ignoring potentially useful complementary mind-body approaches neglects a constellation of therapies that are often simple and effective. I have found that the best approach to cancer is an integrative one, combining the best of modern medicines and technologies with mind-body practices that access our inner pharmacy.

There are currently over 3,500 drugs in our modern pharmacopoeia designed to treat almost every conceivable symptom that can arise in a human being. If each of these drugs performed their intended purpose perfectly, there would probably be little need for, or interest in, alternative medicine. A perfect medicine would be one that completely eliminates the problem it is designed for without any negative side effects. It would need to be taken for only a limited period of time, after which it could be discontinued and the problem would not recur. The drug would not interfere with any other intervention that was being used and would, of course, be inexpensive.

Unfortunately, there are very few medicines that meet these criteria. Drugs that are therapeutically potent often have substantial side effects. This is certainly true for most medicines that are used by patients facing cancer. Whether it is a chemotherapy drug, a narcotic pain reliever, a strong antinausea medicine, a broad-spectrum antibiotic, or a steroid to reduce swelling and inflammation, these pharmaceuticals are powerful weapons that carry risks. This does not mean that you should avoid them; it simply means that they should be used appropriately at the right time and in the right dosage. If mind-body approaches can reduce the need for some medications or reduce the side effects of necessary drugs by activating your internal pharmacy, this is a valuable role for these natural cost-effective interventions.

In the same way that we can fantasize about an ideal drug, we can imagine an optimal complementary approach. It would be fully effective in alleviating the symptom, simple to administer, have lasting efficacy, and be inexpensive. Again, unfortunately, there are few such interventions available. Most mind-body approaches are more effective in gradually relieving chronic concerns than they are in quickly eliminating acute ones. They usually help to reduce, but not completely ease, a symptom, and it often takes repeated efforts until a lasting benefit is obtained. Again, we come back to the concept of using the right tool for the right task. In this chapter, I'll be exploring some common circumstances where mind-body approaches in combination with standard medical care provide the greatest benefit. Let's begin by reviewing the medical approaches that form the mainstay of modern oncology care.

The Modern Medical Cancer Arsenal

Surgery, chemotherapy, and radiation therapy comprise the backbone of modern cancer treatment. Although detractors may refer to these approaches as "slash, trash, and burn," medical treatments have made the difference between life and death for millions of cancer patients. The goal for each of these interventions is basically the same—to separate cancer cells from healthy ones. If this were an easy task, cancer would not evoke the anguish that it does. Unfortunately, the differences between cancer and normal cells tend to be more quantitative than qualitative—cancer cells perform the same functions as normal cells, they just do so more aggressively. Most medical therapies strive to exploit the tendency of malignant cells to grow more rapidly than normal ones. In disrupting the reproductive process, an ideal treatment has a major effect on cancerous tissue but causes minimal injury to normal cells.

Surgery

Surgery is probably the oldest known treatment for the removal of tumors. In the *Sushruta Samhita,* one of the classic ancient Ayurvedic texts dating back 2,500 years, a variety of different surgical procedures are described to extract abnormal masses from the body. The goal of modern cancer surgery is twofold—to confirm the diagnosis and to remove as much malignant tissue as possible. Whenever feasible, the entire tumor is removed. If the cancer is one that is known to travel to lymphatic tissue, several lymph nodes are also usually removed to determine whether the tumor has spread. Even if the entire mass cannot be extracted, reducing the bulk of the tumor load can make other treatments more effective and tip the balance in favor of the person's natural immunity.

If you are scheduled for surgery, prepare for the operation with both body and mind:

~   Follow a simple, healthy diet prior to the procedure, ensuring that you are receiving adequate antioxidant vitamins.
~   Drink plenty of fresh fruit and vegetable juices along with ingesting adequate fiber to ensure that your bowels are moving regularly.
~   Gently massage the anticipated operative area with vitamin E–enriched oil for several days prior to the procedure.
~   Pray and ask those who love you to pray for your rapid and complete recovery.
~   Consider recording a guided meditation exercise to use on the day of the operation. Visualize that the Divine Spirit, in whatever form you conceive it, is acting through the hands of your surgical team.

Radiation Therapy

Radiation therapy dates to the discovery of X rays in 1895 by Marie and Pierre Curie. Today, one-half to two-thirds of people facing cancer receive some form of radiation treatment during the course of their illness. The focused beams of radiation energy are designed to alter the atoms in the DNA of the cancerous cells so that they are no longer capable of reproducing. The science of radiation oncology continues to evolve as ways are discovered to increase the susceptibility of cancer cells to radiation while decreasing the vulnerability of normal cells. Using medications that make tumor cells more sensitive, modifying the dosing schedules, implanting radioactive seeds directly into the malignant tissue, and focusing beams into a radiation "knife" are some of the advances that are improving the efficacy and safety of radiation therapy.

To prepare for your radiation therapy:

~ Visualize the radiation as concentrated light beams, exposing the shadowy nests of renegade cells.
~ Apply soothing, cooling oils, such as coconut or olive, to the skin after each treatment.
~ Although your appetite may be diminished, be certain to eat nutritionally vital foods.
~ Consider taking an adaptogenic herbal nutritional supplement such as ginseng (*Panax ginseng*) or ashwagandha (*Withania somnifera*). A recent study suggested that mice given garlic five days prior to receiving gamma radiation had a reduction in the chromosomal damage to their bone marrow cells, so eating more Italian and Middle Eastern food during your treatments may not be a bad idea.[1]
~ Allow yourself the time to rest each day and create the space to connect with your natural environment on a regular basis.

Chemotherapy

Many people facing cancer have an understandable fear of chemotherapy drugs. Most of these powerful medicines carry powerful side effects, for their toxic impact on cancer cells spills over to healthy cells. If there were equally effective, nontoxic alternatives to chemotherapy, every health care provider treating cancer would gladly embrace them. Although there are steady advances in the development of drugs that enhance our body's ability to fight cancer (biologic response modifiers, or BRMs), the majority of cancer-fighting medications are designed to induce the death of rapidly dividing cells.

Most chemotherapy agents interfere with some aspect of the genetic process. Certain drugs produce breaks in the DNA strands, some interfere with replication of the genetic code, while others prevent the hereditary blueprints from making the essential proteins of the cell. The goal of all chemotherapy regimens is to alter the cancer cells without unduly harming healthy cells. Because of the potency of these medications, cancer specialists have accumulated abundant information about both the success and toxicity of chemotherapy drugs used for most types of cancer. In some malignancies, such as types of leukemia and lymphoma, the medicines are administered with the intention of curing the person of cancer. In other situations, such as certain stages of breast and ovarian cancer, drugs are used in combination with radiation and surgery with the expectation that the cancer can be completely eliminated. In other circumstances, chemotherapy is used to prolong or improve the quality of life in people with cancer but is not anticipated to eliminate all cancer cells from the body.

If it is recommended that you receive chemotherapy as part of your treatment, ask your oncologist the following questions:

1. What are the expectations from the treatment—cure or control?
2. What are the side effects from the medicines?
3. What can be done medically to reduce the side effects?
4. How many courses of chemotherapy are anticipated?
5. How long before you will know if the treatments are effective?
6. How will you be able to evaluate the effectiveness of the treatment?
7. Are there other patients who have received the treatment who would be willing to talk with you?

It is usually helpful to have a friend or family member with you when you are having these discussions with your doctor. Ask them to take notes so you can review the conversation when you return home. Use your finely honed communication skills to express your questions and concerns openly and honestly. Avoid putting your doctors on the defensive, for this usually results in their detailing all possible complications of treatment, even if they are extremely rare. Make your best decision and then prepare yourself to work in concert with your doctor and the medications. As with surgery and radiation, it is important that you provide your body with the nutritional support it will require during your treatment. Perform a daily massage, talk regularly to family and friends, meditate morning and evening, and connect with nature. Consider taking the herb astragalus (*Astragalus membranaceus*), which has been suggested in some, but not all, studies to protect the immune system from the suppressant effects of certain chemotherapy drugs.[2, 3, 4]

Biological Therapies—
The Future of Cancer Treatment?

Recognizing the hazards of potent chemotherapy medications, cancer researchers have sought safer ways to shift the balance of power between the tumor and the host in favor of the person. Although these immune-enhancing approaches have yet to realize their full potential, they are providing some hope that we will eventually have more potent and less toxic treatments available.

There have been some reported successes with anticancer vaccines in patients with malignant melanoma. Proteins derived from tumor cells and made into a vaccine can stimulate the body's immune system to recognize and eliminate runaway cancer cells. Some patients with metastatic malignant melanoma who have undergone vaccine therapy at the University of California San Diego Medical Center have remained healthy years after receiving the therapy.[5]

Another approach to enhancing cancer immunity is the development of antibodies directed at tumor proteins. They are known as monoclonal antibodies, and cancer researchers are designing these tumor-seeking protein missiles to carry tiny chemotherapy or radiation weapons directly to cancer cells, leaving healthy tissues unharmed. Although there are still many hurdles to overcome for these treatments to be clinically practical, scattered reports are beginning to suggest that this innovative approach may be promising.[6, 7]

Finally, there is growing interest in using cytokines to enhance the immune response to cancer. As I discussed in chapter 2, these chemical messenger molecules communicate information between the many different immune cells that are called to respond to a potential invader. Infusing molecules such as interleukin 2 (IL-2) and various interferons are the most commonly used cytokines in cancer therapy, designed to help activate a person's immunity. IL-2 has shown some value in renal cell cancer, and interferon has been used with leukemia and lymphoma. Although they are natural components of our immune system, they do produce side effects when used in high doses.

Coping with Chemotherapy

It is a distinctly human trait that we willingly accept short-term discomfort for the possibility of longer-term benefit. So it is with chemotherapy. We willingly subject ourselves to powerful drugs that carry distressing side effects when we are convinced that their benefits outweigh their risks. Unfortunately, we often compound the direct complications of chemotherapy with emotional and physical distress that is as much self-generated as it is a necessary consequence of the treatment.

Patients receiving chemotherapy experience classical negative conditioning. If ten seconds after a buzzer sounds, we consistently receive an electrical shock, we will soon have a stress reaction each time we hear the buzzer, even before we are shocked. People undergoing cancer treatments often experience three related anticipatory problems: anxiety, nausea, and immune suppression.

> Allison was proud of herself after tolerating her first round of adjuvant chemotherapy for her breast cancer. Although it was not a pleasant experience, she experienced only mild nausea and anxiety. She was, therefore, surprised when the night before her next scheduled treatment, she awoke from a frightening dream in a cold sweat. She was eventually able to fall back asleep but tossed and turned restlessly throughout the night. When in the morning she dragged herself out of bed to get ready for her oncology visit, she became intensely nauseated and light-headed. She finally called her sister to drive her to her appointment, as she did not feel competent to drive herself. Once she received her anti-nausea medicine, her anxiety subsided and she was able to proceed with her treatment course.

The sounds, sensations, sights, and smells of cancer treatment become associated with the side effects of the medicines. A study from the Sloan-Kettering Cancer Center had women drink lemon-lime Kool-Aid while waiting for their chemotherapy infusions.[8] Nurses subsequently visited patients at their homes, offering them a glass of the distinctive green beverage, and found that just the sight of the drink led to an increase in their distress. In addition to the anticipatory anxiety, nausea, and vomiting that many cancer patients experience, there is often impairment in their immune function, even before the chemotherapy medicine is given.[9]

One of the earliest studies that discovered how our interpretation of an experience could influence our immunity was by Dr. Robert Ader over twenty years ago.[10] He exposed laboratory rats to water that was sweetened with saccharin and immediately injected them with cyclophosphamide, a chemotherapy drug that has nausea and vomiting as prominent side effects. Cyclophosphamide is also a potent immune suppressant. The animals vomited as soon as they were given the cyclophosphamide and over the next several days showed the expected suppression in their immune function. Days later, after the rats had recovered, they were again exposed to the saccharin water, and again promptly vomited. This part was not surprising, as it was an example of classical conditioning, not unlike Pavlov training a dog to salivate when he rang a bell. Ader's rodents had been conditioned to vomit when they tasted sweet water.

But something else unexpected was discovered. When the rats were exposed to the saccharin-sweetened water the second time, they again showed a marked suppression in their immune function, even though they had *not* received the cyclophosphamide. Not only had the rats been conditioned to vomit, their immune cells had become conditioned to be suppressed. Their immune cells had learned that sweetened water was harmful to them.

The good news is that we can condition our immune cells to respond positively just as we can condition them negatively. By associating sounds, sensations, sights, smells, and flavors with a life-affirming experience, we can offset the harmful effects of stress on our immune system. In chapter 8 I mention a study from Japan that used aromas to blunt the effects of stress on mice.[11] They were placed in a cage and randomly given distressing, but not life-threatening, electrical shocks. These poor creatures showed rises in levels of stress hormones in their blood and deterioration in their immune system's ability to fight infection. When they were not being tormented, they were allowed to recuperate in a cage that had fragrant cedar wood shavings along with food and water. When the stress procedure was repeated, some of the mice were exposed to the aroma of cedar while they were subjected to the electrical shocks. Despite the same stress as a comparison group of mice, the aroma-exposed critters showed lower levels of stress hormones and insignificant immune changes. Presumably, the memory of safety and comfort associated with the aroma of the cedar shavings blunted the impact of stress.

All of learning is ultimately through association. As newborns we associate the smell of mother with the taste of her sweet milk and produce calming pleasure hormones when she is near. We associate the upsetting sounds of a reprimand (and perhaps a sting on our bottom) with stepping into the street and learn to look both ways before crossing. We associate smiles and praises with high scores on examinations and frowns and restrictions with low scores. Living beings are motivated by the pursuit of pleasure and the avoidance of pain, and we learn to anticipate one or the other by the sensory information that accompanies past feeling. Our internal pharmacy is continuously responding to our interpretations of the world as either nourishing or toxic. With awareness, we can create new associations to generate healing chemicals to aid us in our journey to wholeness.

If you are undergoing chemotherapy, be an active partner in your care, dedicated to maximizing the benefits and minimizing the side effects of treatment:

~ Practice meditation to calm your mind.
~ During chemotherapy, invoke a visualization that interprets the medication as positive and life-affirming.
~ Eat lightly on the day of treatment. Try sipping fresh fruit juices, progressing to soups as your appetite is kindled.
~ Ask a friend or family member to provide a gentle foot or shoulder massage during the treatment.
~ Listen to music that is nourishing or watch a video that is uplifting or humorous.
~ Use an aromatic essential oil to disguise the medicinal smells of the chemotherapy center.
~ Surround yourself with pictures that bring you happiness, comfort, or make you laugh.
~ Share yourself and your stories with other people facing cancer and with the medical staff.

Pain and Suffering

Pain is generally at or near the top of the list of concerns of many people facing cancer. The most common cause of pain is a tumor pressing on or stretching nerves. Other causes of pain in cancer include surgery, certain chemotherapy drugs that are toxic to nerves, and general musculoskeletal discomfort as a result of the tension and reduced mobility associated with cancer and its treatment. Fortunately, there are many effective pain medications available today, ranging from non-narcotic anti-inflammatory medications to oral synthetic opiates to slow-release analgesic patches to potent injectable narcotics. When the right medication is given at the right time, most pain can be well controlled. The challenge is how to achieve maximal pain relief with minimal side effects. The most common adverse reactions to the powerful narcotic pain medications are constipation and mood alterations, particularly drowsiness. Although newer pain relievers have improved the reward-to-risk ratio, the strong analgesics will probably always have some of these undesirable side effects. Therefore, it is worth trying to reduce the need for these powerful weapons against pain, if possible.

> Estelle was struggling with ovarian cancer. Although her doctor was encouraged that the taxol she was receiving was helping, she was exhausted and uncomfortable in her body. She was taking hydromorphone and wearing a fentanyl patch, but she didn't like the feeling of being in a cloud all the time. Her bowels were sluggish, she felt anxious all the time, and she was sleeping poorly.
>
> We agreed to focus on the basics—sleeping, eliminating, and reducing anxiety. She learned meditation and guided visualizations, which provided a temporary respite from her aching. Using diet and natural laxative bowel-enhancing herbs, she was able to reestablish regularity in her elimination. She started gentle yoga practices and made a point to get into bed and wake up earlier. Using these and other mind-body approaches, she was able to move her pain off center stage of her awareness and reduce her need for pain medications by one-third.

We have to distinguish between pain and suffering. The physical sensation of stepping on a tack or putting our foot into a scalding bath is simple enough to understand. Acute pain occurs when a stimulus triggers a pain receptor, which sends the message along nerve fibers from the site of the injury to our brain. In cases where the source of pain is external and avoidable, the pain subsides after a moment or two. It has fulfilled its purpose of instantly getting our attention and making us change what we were doing. Hopefully, as a result of the experience we learned not to repeat the action that caused the unpleasant sensation.

The pain of cancer is different from that of touching a hot stove. The source of discomfort is internal and not so easily escaped. Because you cannot simply avoid the behavior that provokes the pain, the primary sensation extends its territory of influence beyond just a simple reflexive reaction. The pain may cause you to become anxious, irritable, or depressed. If you feel you have no control over the pain, sensations of hopelessness and helplessness arise. The primary uncomfortable sensations of pain have led to an interpretation of suffering.

Most of us at one time or another have had an injury that was a source of pain. While it was healing, the area of discomfort made itself known, but there were times when we completely forgot about the pain. It might be while watching a movie or engrossed in a conversation. We have the capability of at least partially filtering sensory impulses that reach conscious awareness through our attention and our intention. This intrinsic power allows us to separate our interpretation of suffering from the primary sensations.

There are a number of things we can do to mitigate pain. Meditation and visualizations can transport us to a place that is removed from the discomfort. Ask a friend to take you through the following process, reading the instructions in a soft, slow, calm voice. If you find it effective, you can record the script and play it to yourself.

Transcending Pain

~   Allow your eyes to close, take a deep breath, and slowly exhale, allowing your tension to release. As you further relax with every breath, you may notice that your pain calls for your attention. There is no need to resist the sensation. . . . There is no need to fight the pain as you allow the muscles in your shoulders . . . arms . . . and hands to relax. As you continue inhaling and exhaling, the pain requires no effort as you release the tension from your back . . . hips . . . thighs . . . legs . . . and feet. Feel the tightness melt from your neck and head as you begin floating downward through your pain. Allow your awareness to drift through the tension to a quiet place of comfort and relaxation. Enter a space of safety and tranquility in which soft, billowy clouds lazily float by on a warm summer day. The air is perfumed with fragrant flowers and the smell of freshly mowed grass. The gentle, soothing breeze carries the sounds of warbling birds and humming bees as you savor the sensations of comfort and well being. Enjoy this experience of peace and contentment. Allow it to permeate your mind and body. When you are ready, slowly allow yourself to return to this time and place, carrying this experience of ease and serenity back with you.

Choose approaches that help you shift your attention to pleasing thoughts or sensations rather than those focused on the pain. Listen to beautiful music, take a warm bath, get a foot massage, walk along the ocean. Acupuncture and acupressure can be useful tools in taking the edge off uncomfortable sensations. Gentle stretching and yoga postures can facilitate the release of muscle tension. Give yourself the opportunity to laugh heartily and cry freely once a day. Try herbal teas that can take the edge off your anxiety such as valerian, gotu kola, or kava kava. Boswellin, derived from the resin of the tree *Boswellia serrata*, is an Ayurvedic herb with possible anti-inflammatory and analgesic properties that has recently become more widely available in the West. Use your body, mind, and spirit to access that place where pain cannot reach you.

Communicating with Your Doctor

From our earliest childhood days, we want to be comforted when we are injured. If we fall and scrape a knee, there is nothing like Mother's soothing embrace to help us quickly forget our injury. When as adults we encounter illness that causes emotional and physical discomfort, we naturally long for someone to "make it all better." Ideally we are lucky to find a doctor who provides the right blend of comfort and empowerment. Fortunately, most health professionals who choose to enter oncology are compassionate, caring people.

However, unlike dependent children, as adults we have a responsibility to actively participate in our own healing process. We need to ask the pertinent questions and be engaged in the important decisions regarding our care. The key to being an empowered patient is establishing an open line of communication with our health care providers, and it is best to establish the tone of the relationship as early as possible. Use your doctor as an educational resource, providing you with all the information you can digest. Use your doctor as a sounding board to get feedback on information you receive from other sources. Expect to be treated respectfully. If your physician rebukes an approach that seems reasonable to you, ask for a satisfactory explanation. If there seems to be more emotion than reason in the rejection, explain that you are not challenging his or her authority; rather, you simply want to understand how they came to their decision.

More and more physicians are recognizing the value of complementary approaches in healing and are curious to see what value they might provide. Explain to your doctor that you do not want to hide your exploration of other healing modalities, but would like to share your experiences so that you can learn together. Approaching your doctors in a mature, open-hearted manner will almost certainly assure their tolerance, if not actual enthusiasm, for your empowered participation. If despite your best efforts, you feel that the only role your doctor will accept is one of an undisputed authority figure, you will need to make a conscious choice. Either you can accept the role your doctor has defined for both of you and continue your exploration of other healing approaches on your own, or you can choose to find another physician whose style is more flexible. Sometimes the technical expertise of a cancer specialist is such that you are willing to overlook a less than desirable personality. For others, having a doctor from whom you must hide things is unacceptable. It is my deepest wish that you find a doctor who embodies both knowledge of disease and wisdom of life. Such healers are of inestimable value to their patients.

Cancer Therapy Embracing Body, Mind, and Spirit

I like to envision a medical system that embraces the best of the principles discussed in this book. It would not be a disease care system as currently exists, and would not stop at being a health care system. It would be a healing system, dedicated to providing care that honors the sanctity of life and treats each person with dignity, compassion, and love. It would be a place in which each person is treated the way we would want our family members or ourselves to be treated. The very best of standard medical care would be available and always offered in a spirit of caring and respect.

Five years ago I would have thought this model to be a fantasy, not to be realized in my lifetime. Lately there have been some indications that perhaps our collective consciousness is ready to create a genuine healing environment, because we demand and deserve it. I'd like to offer my vision of how a healing cancer center might look if we chose to create one.

The essential essence of a consciousness-based cancer program is the recognition that we are all on a journey together. When one of us stumbles, each of us is affected. The consciousness of the people at our ideal cancer center is the key component of the healing environment. A person with cancer is seen as a precious member of the human community, facing a challenge that all of us will eventually face—our individual mortality.

Genuine compassion and caring permeate the healing environment, and the patient's concerns and convenience are given primary importance.

The environment of the healing center reflects the principle that nourishment is provided through the five senses. As we enter our model cancer center, we are exposed to soothing aromas, calming music, and beautiful, inspiring artwork. Ideally, the treatment rooms look onto a park or other natural setting that is elevating to the spirit. Before receiving any specific therapy, each person is instructed in meditation and visualization techniques associated with the nourishing sounds, smells, and sights. When it is time to begin chemotherapy, a personalized ritual is offered that provides an opportunity for the patient and staff to acknowledge their hopes and fears. If it is consistent with the worldview of the patient, a higher power is invoked to protect and guide the person with cancer and his or her health providers.

Efforts to define the chronobiology of the tumor are made so that the medicines can be given when they are expected to provide the greatest benefit with the least possible risk. While the drugs are administered, the recipient is encouraged to visualize the benefits of the drugs, which are viewed as allies in healing. A gentle massage is provided during the chemotherapy infusion, using essential oils that have been associated with a safe, relaxed state. Encouraging videos and audiotapes are available to watch and listen to while receiving treatments.

Ongoing emotional support groups, educational classes, yoga, and meditation sessions are available to provide inspiration and knowledge. Helpful alternative approaches are readily accessible so the person with cancer is not caught in the middle of a health care ego battle. If despite best efforts the cancer progresses, preparation for a loving, respectful transition is made, with a commitment to quality of life driving every decision.

Although all these components may not be available, cancer centers around the country are exploring many of the above concepts. People facing cancer expect to obtain state-of-the-art medical care for cancer, regardless of which medical center they go to for treatments. Increasingly, patients also want to be treated as human beings who have a disease, rather than as battlefields upon which diseases are fought. As more people expect to be cared for in a way that honors the inherent dignity of humankind, more cancer centers will be implementing innovative ways to mobilize a person's inner healing forces. Then we will have truly holistic healing centers in which the best of mind-body medicine approaches work in concert with the best of Western medical technology. Our collective vision and intent will create these centers of healing.

Commitment to Wholeness

Our bodies are the end products of our experiences and interpretations. To change our bodies, we need to change our experiences. Make a commitment to change your life in the direction of greater love and caring for yourself and those close to you.

1. I commit to using the best of mainstream medicine and complementary approaches to treat my cancer, striving to integrate rather than polarize my healing allies.

2. I commit to communicating with my health care providers openly and honestly. I expect to be treated as an intelligent person, fully capable of participating in the important decisions regarding my care.

3. I commit to helping create a healing cancer center by teaching my health providers what I believe can optimize my journey to wholeness.

CHAPTER 7

Envisioning Wholeness

*Meditation and Creative
Visualization to Enliven Healing*

For the wakeful one whose mind is quiet, whose thoughts are undisturbed, who has relinquished judgment and blame, there is no fear.—BUDDHA, IN THE DHAMMAPADA

You are in your doctor's waiting room and you overhear a nurse telling your doctor there is a problem with your medical chart. You instantly begin to worry, certain that your latest laboratory test showed cause for concern. Your mind starts to race, your heart pounds in your chest, and you feel flushed. You imagine the worst—that after all the treatments you've received, you're going to be told that your cancer is back. You have an impulse to run out of the waiting room and never see another doctor again. You feel angry that at the last visit you were told everything looked fine, and now, in just two months, things have changed. Thoughts dash through your mind, stirring you into an emotional frenzy.

After an interminable wait, you are called into your oncologist's office, bracing yourself for the bad news. He asks you how you're feeling, and you blurt out, "Just tell me what's wrong!" He looks bewildered, asking what makes you think there's a problem. You relate overhearing the nurse's comments, and he chuckles, explaining the "problem" with your chart was that another patient's bill had been filed in it. He reassures you that everything looks fine on your tests and reinforces his expectation that your cancer is behind you.

~

A classical Vedic myth tells the story of a man who felt a prick in his leg while walking along a road. He looked down and glimpsed a snake in a bush. The distraught man instantly panicked and began shouting that a poisonous snake had bitten him. As people rushed to his assistance, he collapsed to the ground, wailing that he didn't want to die. In an effort to help the poor victim, a woman asked where he was walking when bitten, and the nearly delirious man pointed to the side of the road. She rushed over to where he had pointed and discovered a prickly thorn bush. Carefully reaching into it, she pulled out a thick piece of rope, exclaiming that she had found his "snake." Realizing his misunderstanding of the situation, the man's breathing returned to normal, his strength was restored, and everyone in attendance had a good story to tell.

Our minds are thought fields. Our bodies are molecule fields. These two fields are inextricably interwoven so that a disturbance in one generates a disturbance in the other. When we are composed, our thoughts are impulses of balance and creativity and our bodies experience comfort and ease. When we are enduring mental and emotional turbulence, our bodies experience this turmoil as discomfort and agitation. When facing the stress of a serious illness, we compound the anguish in both our bodies and our minds through obsessive thoughts and the corresponding anxiety we feel in our bodies. Each thought triggers emotions that provoke more thoughts and feelings. Often we generate a loop of mind-body turbulence that takes on a life of its own:

"I hope this pain in my back isn't a sign that my cancer is back."
The anxiety results in a lowered pain threshold.

~

"My pain is getting worse. I'm sure it's my cancer."
The discomfort and anxiety lead to a disturbed sleep pattern.

~

"I've been up all night with this pain. It must be my cancer."
The fear results in staying in bed all day, leading to more stiffness.

~

"Now I can barely move without pain."

You see your doctor the next day, and her questioning triggers your memory that you were lifting some heavy boxes the day before the onset of your pain. She makes the proper diagnosis of a simple muscle strain. Within a few days, the discomfort subsides and you regain your equilibrium and optimism.

Interrupting the Cycle

How do we halt these negative spirals of thought and emotion? Anyone who has tried to get to sleep the night before learning the results of an important laboratory test knows how difficult it can be to turn off an active mind. It cannot be accomplished simply by wishing your thoughts would cease and desist. Most of us need a technique to quiet our minds and recapture our state of physical equilibrium. Throughout the ages and around the world, prayer and meditation have served this purpose. When we are able to release control and establish connection with a field that is beyond physical, mental, and emotional boundaries, we are reminded that the localized problem we are facing cannot destroy that which is essential to our nature—our true Self. The mind is a field of ideas, and the body is a field of molecules, but underlying both our minds and bodies is a field of awareness that is unbounded in time or space. The more we are established in this realm of unboundedness, the better we are able to navigate the challenges we face in life.

The process of glimpsing eternity in the midst of timebound awareness may take on different forms for different people. For many, praying to a higher power is the most comfortable approach to go beyond individuality. Whether it is through personal private prayer, reading Holy Scriptures, or attending a religious service in a church, synagogue, temple, or mosque, the ritual of acknowledging the ultimate authority of Spirit over matter has healing power. Dr. Larry Dossey has explored the capacity of prayer to influence recovery from illness, demonstrating that praying can be a powerful and measurable force.[1]

What happens when we pray? First, we shift our attention away from the ruminating thoughts that keep us locked in a cycle of fear and dread, while invoking a force that has meaning and comfort for us. Whether we envision God as a beautiful King of men, a compassionate Divine Mother, a wise, fatherly sage, or a limitless, formless Spirit, opening our heart and mind to the Being beyond all beings enables us to release some measure of fear and replace it with love and trust. The experience of prayer reminds us of other times when we were disheartened, yet we persevered, ultimately gaining valuable experience and knowledge. While praying, our mental turmoil is temporarily subdued and our body is reminded of its natural state of balance, creating a mind-body state that is much more conducive to healing than one of panic and alarm. And of course, if it is compatible with Cosmic Will, our prayers will be answered. I encourage you to pray in whatever form is comfortable, even if it has been a long time since you have done so.

Slipping between the Thoughts

Meditation techniques can encourage a calm and open mind, providing the best opportunity for sending healing messages to our body. There are many effective meditation techniques that provide an expanded state of awareness. By expanded, I mean experiencing more of the unbounded consciousness that underlies the stream of thoughts that occupy our minds. Take a moment, close your eyes, and listen to your internal dialogue. It may sound like this:

> What's the point of listening to my thoughts? . . . I know my thoughts. . . . I've been thinking about how I'm going to pay my doctor bills. . . . When is my next appointment? . . . I think it's next Tuesday. . . . I hope that Nurse Amy is there. . . . She's much nicer than Sharon. . . . Sharon has certainly gained a lot of weight recently. . . . I wonder what my weight is these days. . . . After so many years of trying to lose, I get cancer. . . . Now I'm trying to gain back the ten pounds I lost. . . . I am kind of hungry. . . . I wonder if that frozen pizza is still in the freezer. . . . I really need to defrost that thing. . . .

Meditation techniques are designed to temporarily interrupt the endless conversation that each of us holds with ourselves. During meditation, we are able to experience a state of awareness that is not dependent upon the meaning of the thoughts that occupy our mind. A simple procedure for accomplishing this is through the process of witnessing our breath. Since our breath is a constant accompaniment during every state of consciousness we move through in a day, focusing on our rhythmic pattern of breathing can be a way to transcend the incessant inner dialogue that keeps our minds and bodies activated. Record the following instructions for this breath awareness meditation into a tape player, using a soothing, calming voice. Then play it for yourself, following the instructions with an easy, innocent attitude:

Breathing Awareness Meditation

1. Close your eyes.
2. Take a few slow deep breaths, releasing any tension you are holding with each exhalation.
3. Gently become aware of your breathing.
4. Innocently observe the in and out . . . in and out . . . in and out . . . of your breath.
5. As you are gently witnessing your breath, do not attempt to alter it in any conscious way.
6. As you innocently follow your breath, you may notice that it changes spontaneously. It may become slower and deeper, or it may become faster or shallower. At times your breathing may seem to pause altogether. However your breathing changes, simply allow it to do so. Do not resist any changes in your breathing pattern.
7. As you observe your breath, you will find that at times your attention drifts away to a thought in your mind, a sensation in your body, or a sound in the environment. Whenever you realize that your attention has drifted away from your breath, gently return it back to your breathing.
8. Relinquish any expectation for a particular experience during this time of meditation. Welcome whatever occurs with an attitude of acceptance and innocence.
9. Continue this procedure for about twenty minutes, then allow your attention to float freely for a few minutes before slowly opening your eyes.

During this process, you will probably have moments when you go into a semidrowsy state in which you are awake but having very indistinct thoughts. It may seem reminiscent of the twilight state between sleep and waking that you may experience when dozing on a Sunday morning. Electroencephalographic (EEG) studies have shown this state to be associated with prolonged runs of slower brain patterns known as theta waves, reflecting a gray zone between wakefulness and sleep. This "hypnagogic" state is usually accompanied by a sense of deep physical relaxation as measured by changes in skin resistance, heart rate, and breathing patterns.[2, 3]

Recent studies have suggested that the relaxed state achieved in meditation also may raise levels of melatonin, possibly helping people normalize their sleep/wake cycles.[4]

You may notice brief moments when your mind seems to be completely quiet, yet awake. This is the experience of slipping into the "gap" between thoughts. The Sanskrit term for this experience is *samadhi*, and I would suggest that everybody needs samadhi sometimes.

A less enjoyable experience during meditation is when your mind is filled with thoughts. Every time you bring your attention back to your breathing, you immediately drift off into a train of thinking. This may be accompanied by a sense of physical restlessness. Unlike the experience of the "gap" in which time goes by very quickly, the experience of a very active mind may make a meditation seem interminably long. However, even if your subjective experience is not one of blissful, expanded consciousness, you are gaining benefit from taking time to meditate. I encourage you to continue the practice for the time allocated. You will often notice that just when you are feeling frustrated about how noisy your mind is, you will spontaneously enter a more relaxed and silent space. One of the most important components of successful meditation is not judging the experience but committing the time to look inward, even if it seems rather rowdy on occasion. Although the meditation experience provides value in itself, the greater value is in the stabilizing and centering effect that meditation has on our daily activities.

Using Meditation Instruments

We can go beyond the associative level of thinking using any of the five senses. Listening to chanting, drumming, or uplifting music can have a quieting and expansive influence on our mind. A soothing massage can induce a state of deep relaxation. Gazing at a beautiful sunset, a piece of art, or a spiritual design can temporarily stop the usual chattering of our ordinary thoughts and enable us to experience a state of quiet awareness. In the Vedic tradition, there is a science of how to use the senses to quiet the mind. Because thinking is considered to be a subtle form of hearing, the science of sound is held to be the most direct way to transform the quality of the mind.

Specific vibrations are used to quiet and expand an active mind, caught in a cycle of anxiety and fear. Meditations derived from the Vedic tradition commonly use specific sounds known as *mantras*, the Sanskrit word for "mind instruments." There are hundreds of different mantras that can be used as meditation vehicles. Some of these sacred sounds are taught privately by a teacher during an instruction ceremony. This is the case for Transcendental Meditation (TM) and Primordial Sound Meditation (PSM). These meditation techniques emphasize effortless repetition of a mantra selected for the student by a teacher. In PSM, the mantras are chosen on the basis of a person's birth time and place, according to an ancient system of Vedic mathematics. Bija, or seeds mantras, are used as the objects of internal attention in a similar way that the breath is used during breathing awareness meditation. A person is instructed to gently repeat the mantra mentally, returning to it effortlessly when his or her attention drifts off to thought, sensation, or sound. The primordial sound, which has no real meaning, allows for a temporary interruption in the usual pattern of one meaningful thought's triggering the next. As quieting occurs on the level of mental activity, the body also experiences a deep state of relaxation. Silent mantra meditation techniques are very valuable, and we routinely instruct our patients with cancer in Primordial Sound Meditation at the Chopra Center. Qualified teachers are now available in most major cities in the United States and many countries throughout Latin America, Europe, Asia, Africa, and Australia.

Tantric Meditation

Unlike the mantras used silently in PSM, those derived from the Tantric tradition are often used aloud. Tantra is a beautiful practical spiritual system that seeks to bring spirituality into all facets of life. According to Tantra, there are seven primary energy centers in the body, corresponding to the vital concerns of every human being. Known as *chakras*, or wheels, each center has a particular mantra associated with it, which can be chanted aloud.

The first center is located at the base of the spine and governs basic survival needs. When we are feeling threatened at our core, focusing on and enlivening this energy center can be stabilizing. We will often realize that our fears are out of proportion to the reality we are facing at the present moment.

The second center is located in the area of our reproductive organs and governs our basic sense of connectedness and attractiveness to other human beings. It is responsible for sexuality and procreation. Placing our attention in the second chakra enlivens our basic vital energies.

The third center, localized to the solar plexus, is identified with our ability to fulfill our desires in the world. It is our personal power center, which, when weak, creates a sense of anxiety and impotence. Enlivening this area through attention and intention can help restore our sense of confidence in our ability to accomplish our goals in life.

The fourth center governs our heart, generating our higher human qualities of love, compassion, and empathy. When our heart center is open and healthy, we are comfortable giving and receiving nourishing energy to family, friends, and the people who surround us. When we are feeling isolated, emotionally wounded, or unworthy, putting our attention on our heart chakra can help remind us of our essential connectedness to everyone around us.

The fifth center governs expression and is localized to the throat area. When we are having difficulty expressing our innermost thoughts or emotions, we may feel a sense of restrictiveness in this area. Putting your attention in the area of the throat and consciously releasing any tension you are holding there can provide a sense of both physical and emotional relief.

The sixth center is in the forehead and is associated with insight. Inspiration, knowledge, and understanding are the qualities of this chakra. When life energy is flowing through this center, we comprehend the deeper significance of events in our lives and realize that every step of our journey offers opportunities for expanding wisdom and compassion. It is here that we create and understand the meaning of core-challenging events in our life.

The seventh and final energy center is known as the thousand-petal lotus flower at the top of our head. When this chakra is fully opened, we remember our essence as eternal, unbounded spiritual beings temporarily wrapping ourselves in flesh and bones. This is the center of liberation and enlightenment. The full blossoming of this flower is the ultimate goal of life. Just a taste of the nectar available in this energy center transports us beyond pain and fear.

Each center has a mantra associated with it that can help to release blockages and energize the healing power inherent in the chakra. A simple method of using these mantras is to sit comfortably in an upright posture, close your eyes, visualize the center, take a deep breath, and express the mantra aloud as you exhale. Imagine that the sound is emanating from the center you are envisioning. Say each sound one to seven times, then shift your attention to the next-higher center. When you have gone

Energy Center	Location	Mantra
First	Base of spine	LAM ("A" as in father)
Second	Reproductive organs	VAM
Third	Solar plexus	RAM
Fourth	Heart	YAM
Fifth	Throat	HAM
Sixth	Forehead between eyes	SHAM
Seventh	Top of head	OM ("O" as in home)

through all seven chakras, continue with your eyes closed for several minutes, allowing your attention to be in your body. Many people report they feel a great sense of release and centering as a result of this meditation. I encourage you to try it on your own or with loved ones. If you notice a positive effect, practice this process at least once daily.

I recently witnessed a very positive experience using the chakra mantras in a woman who had been treated for thyroid cancer. Since her surgery, she had complained of a tight feeling in her throat, as if something were subtly restricting her breathing. After an extensive evaluation by her physicians, no organic cause could be identified for her symptom. She was referred to a psychiatrist, but despite several therapy sessions and a trial of an antianxiety medicine, there was no change in her complaint. With the reassurance of an extensive negative diagnostic work-up, I asked this woman to consider her problem in terms of blocked energy. Rather than ascribing her complaint to a structural problem, we explored a subtler approach. She was instructed in the chakra mantras and advised to spend ten minutes a day using the vibrational sound of the fifth center to mobilize energy in her throat. Within just a few days she began to see improvement, and within a month she was no longer troubled by the symptom.

Time and again I have seen the powerful therapeutic value of providing a way for patients to focus their healing energies. I don't know whether there was something specific about the procedure that this woman was taught or whether it simply provided a mechanism for her to mobilize her mental and physical recuperative powers. Regardless of the explanation, the use of a healing mantra is a very cost-effective modality—particularly when it works!

Healing Visualization

Everything in the world can be thought of in terms of energy and information. Energy is the primary substance of the material world, while information is the specific organization of energy into patterns that follow the laws of nature, distinguishing one thing from another. A rose and a daisy are composed of the same basic molecules, but the organization of those molecules generates the obvious differences in form, color, and fragrance.

In our minds, energy and information can be described as attention and intention. Whatever we place our *attention* on increases in importance in our life; when we remove our attention it diminishes in significance. *Intention* is the process of directing the energy of our awareness in specific channels to achieve a desired effect.

Shifting our awareness from one object to another is the process of directing our attention, the localizing value of consciousness. We allow into consciousness only that which captures our attention. An airplane may be flying overhead while we are reading an engrossing novel, but it may never register in our conscious awareness. Although you may be wearing a watch on your wrist right now, until you shift your attention to it, it is filtered from your awareness. The more attention we place on something, the greater influence it has in our lives. If I focus on weight training, my bulging muscles will reflect the increased attention I am placing on bodybuilding. If I focus on a pain in my body, the discomfort will consume more of my life. If I focus on healing my body, mind, and emotions, I will see transformations in these aspects of my life.

Intention is the process of directing attention for a specific purpose. The same action with different intentions will have very different outcomes. Calling your dog with the intention of punishing him for getting into the garbage will have a different effect from calling him to feed him. Calling a person with the intention of selling something has a different effect from approaching someone and offering a charitable donation.

When facing an illness, we can use our attention and intention to direct our healing response to the area that requires care. Focusing our attention on a part of our body with the intention of bringing healing energy to that area will have a different effect from envisioning the area with the expectation of pain. Attention alone has healing power; when activated with consciously directed intention, it can be even more powerful.

Creative visualization is a powerful way to use the power of attention and intention to mobilize our inner healer.

There are many different techniques of guided imagery and visualization. Although visualization has been a part of healing traditions for thousands of years, O. Carl Simonton pioneered the use of guided imagery for people facing cancer in the United States in the 1970s.[5] Early practices focused on invigorating immune cells by imagining a battleground in which cancer cells are alien invaders and the immune system is a defending army. Such an approach can be empowering, although this conflict-laden imagery can sometimes lead to battle fatigue.

Increasingly, visualization approaches oriented toward invoking harmonizing images are being favored. Rather than generating combat mentality, imagery can be used to calm an inner environment of distress and encourage a healing response. I have found that it can be helpful to see malignant cells as disoriented and confused entities. Having forgotten their intended purpose, these renegade cells have lost their meaning in life. This framing of cancer opens the possibility of reestablishing balance by reminding the wayward cells of their legitimate reason for existence.

A beautiful concept of Vedic wisdom has something valuable to offer in this context. The principle of *dharma* holds that each human being has a unique purpose in life. When a person is living his or her dharma, he or she can express a unique talent while serving others. In a parallel way, each cell in our body has a dharma that is expressed when the cell is performing its specific role while serving the entire mind-body physiology. A cancer cell, having forgotten its dharma, is no longer able to serve the body. Clearing the blockages to the free flow of energy and information and allowing loving nourishment to circulate creates the possibility of restoring of the memory of wholeness.

Visualizing a healthy functioning body is one way to encourage this memory of health. Try recording your reading of the following visualization and listening to it after a meditation when your awareness is settled in the quiet field of pure potentiality. This process uses attention and intention to enliven your inner healer.

Healing Visualization

~   Sit comfortably, close your eyes, and take a deep breath. Now, slowly exhale, allowing the tension in your chest, shoulders, and abdomen to release. Innocently observing your breath, allow each exhalation to take you to a quieter, more comfortable, more relaxed state. Release the tension, the tightness, and the weight of your body with each breath.

~ Envision or imagine that you are in a beautiful, serene natural environment. The air is warm, the sun is shining, the sky is clear, and the ground is covered with sweetly fragrant, soft grass. Find a comfortable spot and lie down in the grass, allowing the earth to cradle you. Feel the soothing sun on your body. Enjoy this time of peace and serenity.

~ Now envision your body as a glowing cocoon of golden light. See and feel the life force radiating within and around you. Notice the area of your body that is unwell. See the ailing cells as shadowy beings that have lost their way. They have forgotten their dharma, their purpose in life, and in their effort to gain attention, they have gone beyond their healthy boundaries.

~ Now imagine that a warm, pure, healing light is gradually glowing brighter in your heart. Allow it to radiate comfort, peace, and love throughout your entire body, encompassing every cell. As the soothing, healing light fills your being, direct its luminescence to the area of illness. Allow the purifying light to illuminate the shadows hiding there and watch them melt away. Observe the clearing of darkness as the healing energy perfuses the tissues, bringing lightness and clarity.

~ Allow the nourishing energy of the environment—the pure air, the nurturing earth, the luminous sun—to infuse your being, purifying and nourishing your body, mind, and soul. Release the resistance, release the pain, release the fear. In the light and warmth of your healing awareness, and with the wisdom of Nature, the memory of wholeness is rekindled.

Personalize your visualization, invoking imagery that you find healing and empowering. I have found it valuable for cancer patients to write out scripts for various possible scenarios. Below is a suggested guided visualization to use while undergoing chemotherapy. Make a recording and listen to it through headphones while you are receiving your treatments.

Chemotherapy Visualization

~ I am in my sacred space on top of my healing mountain. The sky is deep blue and the warm gentle breeze is embracing me in a cocoon of healing energy. Celestial beings of light and love surround me, sending me encouragement, caring, and strength. With each breath, I inhale the sweet fragrance of vitalizing flowers, soothing and nourishing my body, mind, and soul. I feel infused with trust and hope, secure that a profoundly wise and healing force is guiding me. I see the chemotherapy medicine as a gift from Nature's inner sanctum, a nectar of healing. As the medicine is infused into my vein, I envision it as a golden stream seeking out cells that have become distorted and gently encouraging them to sleep. My healthy cells recognize their need for assistance in reestablishing balance, honoring and appreciating the powerful medicine I am receiving. I know at the core of my being that the alliance of this essential medicine with my innate recuperative powers is creating the optimal environment for healing.

I have observed this visualization shift a person's entire perspective on a chemotherapy regimen. A person undergoing a demanding treatment for cancer may regress and begin to feel like a passive child being forced to undergo therapy by an authority figure. Eliciting an empowering image as suggested in the chemotherapy visualization assists the person in recapturing their sense of partnership and choice in their own treatment. I believe that we will be able to show that these approaches can measurably help to reduce the side effects and enhance the benefits of harsh but beneficial cancer treatments.

Visualizations can be created for daily use during and following your cancer therapy. You can create a calming visualization to be listened to at night when your mind is trying to settle down. You can use imagery to improve your energy level when fatigue seems to be overwhelming. You can use visualizations to reduce anxiety. Be creative, using as many of the senses as you can to create a multisensory healing experience. If there is someone in your life who has always provided encouragement and support for you—a family member, friend, health provider, therapist, or member of the clergy—ask that person to record a message for you that provides the nurturing influence you need. Think about what effect you would like to create, then envision the scene that will support the intended outcome. Always spend at least ten minutes quieting your mind with breathing awareness or a mantra meditation procedure before starting your imagery. A calm and centered awareness provides the best inner environment to cultivate a specific healing response. Your imagination can be a powerful ally in your healing journey.

Commitment to Wholeness

Our bodies are the end products of our experiences and interpretations. To change our bodies, we need to change our experiences. Make a commitment to change your life in the direction of greater love and caring for yourself and those close to you.

1. I will take the time to meditate each day, accessing my inner field of silence, creativity, and healing.

2. I will utilize creative visualizations to enliven my inner healer on a regular basis, understanding that attention and intention are the primary forces of the universe.

3. I will use visualizations to create a sense of safety and empowerment during my therapeutic regimens.

CHAPTER 8

Sensual Healing

*Using Sound, Touch, Sight, and Smell to
Awaken Our Inner Pharmacy*

We live on the leash of our senses.—DIANE ACKERMAN

Amy was feeling sick to her stomach as she prepared for her visit to her oncologist. She thought her nausea was under control, but as the image of Bay General Hospital loomed in front of her, she began feeling queasier. Walking into the lobby, she was assaulted by the sounds of doctors being paged, gurneys rolling by, and intense conversations taking place in hallways. Exiting the elevator to the oncology floor, she caught a whiff of the antiseptic disinfectant used on the chemotherapy unit. A wave of nausea came over her, causing her to retch. The sounds, sights, and smells of the hospital were inextricably interwoven with her past experience of treatment.

How do we learn about life? We ingest the world around us through our five senses, make an interpretation, pass judgment on the experience, and store access to the information in the networks of our brain. Life education begins long before we pass through the birth canal with large chunks of preconceptions carried on our DNA molecules. By the second trimester, we are capable of receiving and recording experiences that filter to us through our watery inner space capsule. A fetus can perceive sounds, sensations, light, and even taste, providing the unborn child with a hazy but increasingly rich picture of the world.

Early perceptions shape our later ones. If you were raised with dogs, seeing a new puppy, hearing its yelping, feeling its soft fur, and smelling its distinctive breath will trigger joyful childhood memories. If, however, your earliest canine encounter was with your neighbor's aggressive pooch, whose ferocious barking regularly frightened you, even an awkward, squirming pup might elicit fear and anxiety in you.

Every species, every culture, and each individual flavors reality with preconceptions and interpretations based upon history. Within a given community, specific expectations become the template for reality; if something falls outside of the template, it is disregarded or ignored. An American may look upon an eel in an aquarium with fascination. A Japanese person may look at the same animal and see it as a culinary treat. Rock and roll music may be musical nectar to a baby boomer but may sound like agitating noise to a native of the Middle East. Even within a culture, individuals have widely varying tastes as to which sensory experiences are nourishing and which are toxic. Go to a movie with your friends, and invariably some will find it wonderful while others will be bored. As great Western scientists and the timeless wisdom traditions tell us, reality is not fixed and absolute; rather, it is a process of perception and interpretation. I once heard this succinctly expressed as "Reality— what a concept!"

Our minds and our bodies are inextricably linked. Every impulse that engages the mind has a corresponding fluctuation in the body. Every mood, emotion, recognition, insight, and idea simultaneously generates a change in the chemistry or electrical activity within our brains. These subtle variations are communicated to the rest of the body through chemical messengers that inform the heart, gut, lungs, and immune cells as to our state of mind. Although we usually think of intelligence as being localized to the nervous system, in actuality intelligence is present in every cell in our body. One measure of intelligence is the ability to make optimal choices in response to changes in our environment, and every healthy cell in our body meets this criterion. Whether we are talking about an islet cell in our pancreas calculating the precise amount of insulin to release, an immune cell determining how aggressive to be with a pollen spore, or a kidney cell deciding how much sodium to absorb, intelligence permeates our body.

If we accept that our cumulative experiences generate the molecules that structure our bodies, we can begin to understand that changing our perceptions and interpretations can change our quality of life. Imagine that the only sounds you heard day and night were car alarms, arguments, and gunshots. Contrast that experience with living next to a melodious brook, rich with the sounds of warbling birds and virile bullfrogs. Imagine the differences in your daily quality of life if you lived downwind of a garbage dump versus next to a botanical garden. Our sensory perceptions subtly yet powerfully craft our reality map. Changing our inputs can transform our reality.

Healing Harmonics

In the beginning was the Word, and the Word was with God and the Word was God. . . . and the Word was made flesh and dwelt among us.
JOHN 1:1, 14

Sound is the stirring of silence. The vibration of air is intimately connected with life. Thought is consciousness in motion, breath is air in motion, and speech is breath in motion. We swim in a sea of vibration through which we perceive the motion of the world around us. Pause for a moment and attend to the sounds around you. Hear the conversations, background music, footsteps, passing cars, and droning airplanes that usually go unnoticed but provide the backdrop for our conscious communication. The increasing noise pollution that is a constant feature of our urban landscape causes a subtle but tangible erosion in our sense of well being. Consciously changing the quality of sound we are exposed to in our environment can noticeably enhance our quality of life.

Directed human sound has been a powerful force throughout the story of humankind. Our earliest efforts at using sound therapeutically were probably intended to imitate the vibrations of Nature in hopes of invoking her healing energy. Early medicine men beat on animal skins stretched over tree stumps, eliciting a trance with their rhythmic cadence. Despite our technological sophistication, most of us experience the same hypnotic response to drumming as our ancient ancestors, perhaps because it reminds us of our earliest auditory memory—the sound of our mother's heartbeat while floating in her watery womb. Early musicians sought to emulate the wind through flutes and reeds, and few of us today can resist the transporting effect of enchanting flute music. There is something primordial about the sound of air vibrating within a tube, and most of us in our past have taken some delight in puffing on a recorder or blowing across the mouth of a Coke bottle. The next step in our musical evolution probably occurred as we stretched dried strips of sinew tightly across resonant hollow branches, developing new possibilities for harmonic vibrations. Early musicians certainly would have noticed that changing the tension and length of the cords on these primitive string instruments evoked a wide range of emotional responses, as do guitars, violins, and cellos today.

Our nearest, but not necessarily simplest, instrument for sound is our own vocal apparatus, capable of producing a wide repertoire of vibrations from whistling to chanting to language. Although we place a high premium on the precision of our words, studies have suggested that more than a third of human communication is through the tone of our voice, with less than 10 percent reflecting the sophistication of our vocabulary.[1] Most of us have heard from our mothers, "It's not what you say, it's how you say it that counts." I wish that more health care providers would heed this sage advice.

Human sounds can incite or subdue us. We may not consciously recall the lullabies our mother sang to us as an infant, but we continue to pass down these sweet, soothing melodies from generation to generation. Dynamic military marches have mobilized armies for centuries, and the Bible reminds us of the power of sound in the story of Joshua and his tribe, who were able to topple the walls of Jericho with a few trumpets and a lot of shouting. From the sound of chalk screeching across a blackboard to the cooing of mourning doves at dawn, we intuitively understand that sounds can provide toxicity or nourishment to our body, mind, and soul, depending upon the quality of the vibration.

Using Sound to Heal

There is a new recognition of the potential therapeutic benefit of sound in health care, and although the start has been languid, momentum is picking up. Music therapy is being used in a wide range of clinical settings with inspiring results. Relaxing music offered to patients after major surgery reduces anxiety and leads to lower requirements for pain medications.[2] Patients who watch relaxing music videos after open heart surgery have less discomfort and sleep better.[3] Newborn babies in neonatal units, elderly folks with depression or memory loss, patients with strokes and Parkinson's disease, and healthy athletes all benefit from exposure to the melodies and rhythms of music.[4-10] Closer to home, music can reduce anxiety and the side effects of chemotherapy in children and adults facing cancer.[11, 12]

How do we use this sound information to enhance the healing process? I believe the most important factor is to choose vibrations that resonate with your body, mind, and soul. Recently, a delightful lady facing breast cancer told me somewhat sheepishly that she thought she ought to listen to ethereal New Age music when receiving chemotherapy, but that she really wanted to hear some great B. B. King jazz. She went with the jazz and found it inspiring to imagine that her chemotherapy was rousing her immune system like a band stirring up the crowd on New Orleans' Bourbon Street at Mardi Gras.

Nature Sounds

There are almost unlimited ways in which we can use sound to enliven our healing power. Some of the most nourishing sounds for many people are the natural vibrations of nature. We can assess our disconnection with our natural environment in terms of how far or long we have to travel before we can hear sounds produced only by nature. In some towns, you can spend time in your backyard without noticeable intrusion, but in many major urban centers, people must travel hours before they can escape the cacophony of civilization.

Visit nature regularly and absorb the sounds that surround you. Listen to the wind moving through the leaves, hear the breathing of the ocean as it crashes against the shoreline, ingest the calls of seagulls. On a warm summer night, listen to the rumble of thunder in the distance and notice the chirping of the crickets, the humming of the cicadas, the hooting of the owls. There is a symphony of sounds in our natural environment, upon which we are welcome to eavesdrop whenever our internal or external noise level subsides.

If we cannot directly access these sounds, there are many wonderful recordings of natural environments available. The chatter of monkeys in a tropical rain forest, the mating bellows of humpback whales, and the calls of whooping cranes are as close as your tape or CD player. Create your selection of nature sounds and use them to remind you that human beings are part of a large, diverse ecology, governed by unfathomable wisdom.

Chanting

Melodic intonations intended to create a sacred experience have been a part of spiritual traditions for thousands of years. Chanting prayers or the sacred names of God creates an expansive and harmonizing effect in both those who are chanting and those who listen to the chants. There has been a recent resurgence in the appreciation of Gregorian chanting, which dates to the Middle Ages.[13] These beautiful songs, sung in unison, elevate our awareness and nourish our hearts with their purity and beauty.

Gregorian chants are derived from the traditional Jewish chanting of prayers that go back thousands of years. Continuing an age-old tradition, modern-day thirteen-year-old boys and girls repeat the traditional melodies and words during their Bar and Bat Mitzvah ceremonies, their ritualized initiation into the community of responsible adults.

Brahmin priests in India spend years memorizing the timeless chants of the Vedas, recounting the process of creation and invoking the forces of nature. Even without understanding the Sanskrit words, listeners are transported to primordial states of being as these fundamental vibrations resonate at deep levels of awareness. A similar effect occurs while listening to Tibetan Buddhist chanting. The resonant mantras of Vedic and Buddhist chants create a resonance that harmonizes body, mind, and spirit in those that experience these ancient tones.

You can have a taste of this effect through a simple procedure. The vowel sounds of every alphabet are primary vibrations that can have a calming influence when toned. Sitting comfortably, take a deep breath and, with your exhalation, tone the sound "ahhhh." Notice the centering influence this sound has on you. Repeat the procedure, this time toning the sound "eeeee." Notice that this vowel has a more localizing effect, creating a vibration in the roof of your mouth and in your sinuses. Proceed through the rest of the vowels, "iiiii," "ooooo," and "uuuuu," noticing the pleasant sensations that are created as well as the subtle differences with each sound.

Try listening to these ancient beautiful sacred songs, innocently experiencing their healing power. You will notice how effortlessly they help connect you with the timeless wisdom traditions from which they derive. Create a healing environment through these sounds in your home, car, and workplace. I provide a list of my favorite choices in the references for this chapter.

Music

Any music can be healing if it inspires, relaxes, encourages, or creates enthusiasm for life in you. Music can be a valuable tool to access our deeper emotions, as it is our most heartening nonverbal form of communication.

Music can serve as a vehicle to delve into feelings that we need to bring into our awareness to heal and release.

The richness of classical music provides a valuable medium for many people to universalize their emotional challenges. Listening to Vivaldi's *Four Seasons*, Beethoven's *Emperor Concerto*, Bach's *Jesu, Joy of Man's Desiring*, or Mozart's *Flute Concerto* opens our hearts, reminding us of our special place in this vast cosmos. Regardless of the challenge we are facing, powerful music can allow us to transcend our localized perspective and glimpse the greater meaning. Take the time to listen to the timeless vibrations of Western culture, which have thrived over centuries because of their universal appeal.

There has been a blossoming of music composed by modern musicians specifically designed to relax and mobilize healing images. Many of these beautiful harmonic journeys can be used to reduce anxiety and help you fall asleep. A list of my favorites is included in the reference section for this chapter. Explore on your own, choosing selections that resonate with your spirit.

Therapeutic Music

If you experience the power of music as something tangible in your life, there are ways to maximize its potential benefits. Music has traditionally been used to add texture to a meaningful ritual. Whether it is the inauguration of a new American president, a school pep rally, graduation from college, a wedding procession, or a religious ceremony, music can add another dimension to the experience, deepening its impact on our body, heart, and soul. The more of our senses an experience engages, the more vibrant the memory will be created in our awareness.

We can use sound and music to engender a positive life-supporting association between an experience and a healing response. Choose or create a guided visualization and select music that you find beautiful and heartfelt to accompany it. Then use it at times when you seek to enter a healing state. For example, prior to beginning chemotherapy treatments, create your guided meditation and then use it only during your treatments. Another possibility is to play your musical selection during a wonderful therapeutic massage. When you use the same musical piece during treatment, you will trigger the memory of the deep relaxation you felt during your body treatment. If you have a good relationship with your oncologist, ask him or her to record a few minutes of encouraging words to which you can overlay a musical tract. Listening to your doctor's reassuring voice while you are receiving the treatments he or she has recommended can provide deep levels of healing nourishment. A study looking at this approach shows that it can substantially reduce anxiety.[14]

Healing Words

One of the most important, and unfortunately most neglected, aspects of the effect of sound on healing is the language that we use to convey information about illness. In a moment, we can convert hope into despair and vice versa. I am dismayed at how often I hear people with cancer describe the way they were given information about their illness. At times, they felt assaulted by information that was provided in such a demoralizing way that they could not absorb any further details. A simple shift in the use of language can make a big difference on the impact words have on a person's mind-body system. Saying that someone has a 25 percent chance of dying from his or her illness over the next five years can be easily reframed as a three-in-four chance of overcoming the cancer. Even if the statistics are less optimistic, it is critical that both health care providers and patients remember that there are many people who beat the average odds. Science has, to date, spent little effort exploring the reasons why some people have exceptional outcomes in a variety of serious illnesses. Benjamin Disraeli once said, "There are three kinds of lies: lies, damned lies, and statistics." We have to remember that statistics apply to groups, not individuals. If the median annual income in La Jolla, California, is fifty thousand dollars, it doesn't help me if I am making minimum wage. Similarly, it doesn't faze me if I am earning one hundred thousand dollars a year to know that the average person is making less. It is essential not to allow yourself to become discouraged by statistical information. Use numbers to make intelligent choices, but do not allow the numbers to use you. Talk to your health care provider about your desire to receive information and your expectation that it will be offered with compassion and hope. This is an inherent right of every human being.

Balancing Mind and Body with Sound

In chapter 3, I introduced the Ayurvedic principles of movement, transformation, and structure and discussed how different foods can have predictable effects on these physiological forces. We can consider the influence of input from all of our senses in a manner similar to the way in which we perceive the effect of food on our mental and physical states. Sounds can be classified and utilized according to their tendency to pacify the wind, fire, or earth elements in our systems. If you are having trouble sleeping at night because your mind is racing, this excessive *wind* can be pacified with soothing, harmonious sounds. A Brahms lullaby, a resonant Gregorian chant, the sounds of a distant thunderstorm, or the deep bellowing of whales all have the effect of quieting our mental clamor. If the *fire* in your system is aggravated and you are feeling frustrated and irritated, music that is sweet and calming will cool your rankled mood. Enchanting flute sounds, heartfelt acoustic guitar music, some cool jazz, or the flowing sounds of moving water seem to have the inherent capacity to soothe our savage breast. If the *earth* force has accumulated excessively in your system and you are feeling dull and lethargic, listen to vibrations that will awaken your soul—an old Rolling Stones or Bob Seger song, some driving drum sounds, Handel's *Royal Fireworks Music*, or the roaring of lions on an African savanna. I have found that the best way to use music therapeutically is not to intellectualize the process, but rather, go to a music store and listen to samples, feeling the influence they have on your heart and soul, body and mind.

Healing Touch

One touch of nature makes the whole world kin.
WILLIAM SHAKESPEARE

If soul may look and body touch,
Which is the more blest?
WILLIAM BUTLER YEATS

Stanley James had been admitted three times in six weeks to the hospital since his original surgery for a cancerous colon polyp. Although every indication pointed to a complete removal of the malignancy, his abdominal wound was healing poorly. The original incision had opened, and he was again requiring intravenous antibiotics for an infection. His mild diabetes was well controlled with insulin, but his recuperative powers seemed weakened. When I spoke with Mr. James, I learned that he had no family support and was trying to recover at home with daily visits by a home health nurse. He was not eating or sleeping well and was feeling quite depressed. Although all these underlying deficiencies were contributing to his sluggish healing, the issue that seemed most distressing to me was the fact that this poor man had not been lovingly touched for years. In fact, other than the inspection of his surgical site, *Mr. James wasn't touched at all.*

I arranged for a physical therapist to perform limited massages during her range-of-motion session with Mr. James (therapeutic massages are not covered by most insurance companies). At first he seemed barely capable of perceiving the nourishing tactile sensations, but after several sessions, the patient reported a growing sense of welcome relaxation and well being. A body therapist began providing regular massages for him when he was discharged home, and within several weeks, his incision was on its way to full recovery.

What role did therapeutic touch play in his healing? As a scientist, I cannot give you a definitive answer. As a doctor and a human being I would agree with Mr. James's belief that being touched in a loving and compassionate way was an essential ingredient in his recovery.

When we utter expressions like "Your music really touched me" or "I felt hurt by his sarcastic remarks," we are intuitively acknowledging the translation of sound into touch. Touch is vibration perceived through our skin, and like sound, the quality of the tactile vibration determines whether the sensation is pleasurable or painful, nourishing or toxic. The difference between a caress and a slap is a function of the energy and information carried in the impression. A slap on the back by an old college buddy will feel vastly different and elicit a response dramatically distinct from one by an irate fan of an opposing football team. The tender stroke of your beloved may elicit pleasure and relaxation, while a premature caress on a first date may eliminate any possibility of further encounters.

Our skin is the physical boundary between our environment and ourselves. Our experience of this boundary is basic to our feelings of being safe or threatened, nurtured or neglected. Studies in infant animals have shown us how critical touch is to normal development. Deprive a baby monkey of its mother's fondling, and the infant will lack normal social skills and be more susceptible to illness. We have learned that the skin is not simply a protective barrier between our inner and outer environments, but a rich and dynamic organ system, replete with growth-promoting factors, natural pain chemicals, immune modulators, and transmitter molecules.

Studies on the healing potential of therapeutic touch are steadily expanding. Early reports in the 1980s showed the benefits of providing "kinesthetic tactile stimulation" to premature infants.[15] We now know that babies born to HIV-positive mothers, infants exposed to cocaine, and newborns with serious medical problems all benefit from regular loving touch.[16, 17] As every parent intimately understands, having a new baby is inexpressibly joyful and unbelievably exhausting. The stresses associated with a newborn are magnified in teenage mothers, whose abilities to care for themselves and their babies may be severely challenged. Providing adolescent moms with a brief massage twice a week reduces their anxiety and lowers the levels of stress hormones circulating in their bodies.[18]

Our new model of healing recognizes that intelligence is in every cell of the body. Our skin is not only our largest organ but contains a vast pharmacy of healing chemicals. Recall how you feel after a therapeutic massage or loving caress from your spouse. Your mind becomes quieter, you may feel so relaxed that you can easily fall asleep, any pain or tension you have been carrying in your body subsides, and you experience a sense of comfort, safety, and well being. These sensations are a result of powerful natural chemicals that are released or stimulated as a result of being touched. If while at work you receive a fifteen-minute shoulder rub, not only will you probably take fewer days off but your blood pressure will be lower.[19] If you are a patient in an intensive care unit, massage can be used to reduce anxiety, lower pain, and even stabilize your heart rhythm.[20, 21] Another way of describing these effects is to say that loving touch generates antianxiety medications, pain relievers, and heart rhythm stabilizing medicines. The beauty of massage is that it accesses our inner pharmacy in such a way that all the side effects are positive.

Enhancing Immunity, Relieving Pain

There are two very direct benefits of massage for people facing cancer: immune stimulation and pain relief. A small number of studies have suggested that therapeutic touch can enhance our immune function. A simple ten-minute back rub has been shown to not only reduce anxiety but to actually increase our secretion of infection-fighting antibodies.[22] Men infected with the AIDS virus who receive massage show a number of positive changes in their immune function. Their natural killer cells increase in number and ferocity, as do other immune cells involved in fighting infection and cancer.[23] The implications for cancer are important because natural killer cells are important in eliminating circulating cancer cells before they have the opportunity to find a place to grow.

Pain is one of the greatest fears of every person facing cancer. Fortunately, modern medicine has many powerful pain-relieving drugs that are being increasingly refined to reduce their side effects and increase their potency. Still, most people with cancer wish to reduce their need for narcotic medications as much as possible, and it is here that massage has some meaningful benefits to offer.

Pain and anxiety are closely linked. We often compound our suffering by worrying about pain that may be approaching even if we are comfortable in the moment. Reducing stress through massage has a prompt benefit in reducing our apprehension about anticipated pain. I commonly see people facing cancer who are so afraid of perceiving their body that they imagine it only as a source of discomfort. Therapeutic touch provides a different experience, rekindling the memory of our body as a source of pleasure and enjoyment. This invigorates our internal pain-relieving system to produce those essential chemicals, the endorphins that are more powerful than any pharmaceutical analgesic. Imagine this conversation between your mind and your body:

BODY: I am feeling really sore today. I've barely recovered from surgery, and now I have to go in every day for radiation treatments.
MIND: I am so tired of this cancer business. I'm scared that it's never going to end and this pain will keep getting worse.
BODY: Ouch! Just rolling over in bed is painful. I don't see how I can possibly tolerate any more treatments.
MIND: This really is too much. All I want to do is sleep. At least then I don't have to listen to my body.

A wise and compassionate friend calls to tell you she is sending over a massage therapist, skilled in caring for people with cancer.

BODY: This massage feels wonderful. I didn't realize how much tension I have been holding in my shoulders.
MIND: Finally, my body is sending me messages other than of stress and discomfort. My endorphin production plant is starting to kick in again.

BODY: My circulation is improving from this stroking, and I am actually beginning to feel alive for the first time in weeks.

MIND: What a relief to know that I can experience some basic enjoyment. I'm feeling hopeful again and have decided to do everything I can, from within and without, to improve my chances of successfully overcoming this illness.

It's funny how changes in technology lead to changes in worldviews. When the stethoscope was first introduced into clinical medicine in the 1800s, there was heated debate as to how the device would create a physical barrier between the doctor and the patient. There was genuine concern that the stethoscope would diminish the therapeutic value of the doctor's putting his ear on the skin of the patient. Since that time, there has been steady erosion in the use of touch to diagnose and heal. Fortunately, we are again recognizing the benefits of touching each other with compassion, sensitivity, and love. Several recent reports have suggested that therapeutic touch can significantly complement pharmaceutical agents in relieving the emotional and physical suffering of cancer.[24, 25]

Practicing Healing Touch

It would be great if we could receive a massage each day from a professional therapist. Although this is not feasible for most of us, we can still profoundly benefit from the healing benefits of touch on a daily basis. First, encourage your family and friends to touch you more. A shoulder rub, a gentle hand massage, or a sensitive foot shiatsu treatment do not require professional training and can still feel great. Just holding hands while watching a movie or taking a walk can provide the nurturing benefit of touch. Americans have ambivalent feelings about touching, for which we pay a price. Certain Latin American cultures are more comfortable expressing themselves tactually and do not place such a stigma on touching as we do in the United States. Touch, and allow yourself to be touched by, those you love, and your immune cells will thank you.

The self-massage, derived from the Ayurvedic tradition, is a wonderful way to enhance well being. It can be performed on a daily basis and offers most of the benefits of a professional treatment. It can be adapted to your time schedule, taking as long as fifteen minutes or as little as a few. It is generally performed before taking a bath or shower, which can be in the morning or evening. If you tend to feel sluggish first thing in the morning, a self-massage can be invigorating and enlivening. If you are having trouble turning off your mind at night, a massage followed by a warm bath can be calming and soothing.

The choice of oil used can add a subtle healing benefit. Just as every food can be characterized according to its ability to influence the wind, fire, or earth element in our mind-body system, so can massage oils. Different oils have been traditionally used to balance the appropriate element. If you are feeling ungrounded with anxiety or insomnia, use a heavier, warmer oil such as sesame or almond, applied with gentle strokes. If you are feeling overheated, irritable, and cranky, try using a lubricant with more cooling properties, such as coconut or olive oil. If you are feeling heavy, congested, and lethargic, try a hotter, lighter oil such as sunflower, safflower, or mustard seed. People with an abundance of earth in their physiology usually prefer deeper, vigorous massages. If you feel you are carrying too much weight, you can also perform the self-massage procedure with a dry silk or linen glove. It will have a stimulating effect, increasing circulation while defoliating the top layer of dead skin cells.

Preparing for the Massage

~ Before it is used, oil should be cured once by slow and careful heating in a glass or metal pot. Place a few drops of water in the oil and remove the pot from the heat as soon as the water boils out of the oil. *The oil must be watched carefully while heating to prevent a fire.* Just before beginning the massage, a small quantity of oil can be gently reheated by placing it in a plastic squeeze bottle, which is then warmed under hot tap water.

Full Body Massage (5–10 minutes)

~ Begin by pouring a tablespoon of warm oil onto the scalp. Using mainly the flat of the hand, massage the oil in vigorously. Cover the entire scalp with small circular strokes, as if shampooing. Move to the face and ears, massaging more gently. Gentle massage of the temples and backs of the ears is especially good for settling the air element.

~ Using both the flat of the hand and the fingers, massage a small amount of oil onto the neck, front and back, and then the shoulders. Vigorously massage the arms, using a circular motion at the shoulders and elbows, and long back-and-forth motions on the upper arms and forearms.

~ Avoid being excessively vigorous on the trunk. Using large, gentle circular motions, massage the chest, stomach, and lower abdomen. Ayurveda traditionally advises moving in a clockwise direction. A straight up-and-down motion can be used over the breastbone.

~ After applying a bit of oil to both hands, gently reach around to massage the back and spine as best you can. Use an up-and-down motion. As with the arms, vigorously massage the legs with a circular motion at the ankles and knees, straight back-and-forth on the long parts. Use whatever oil remains to vigorously massage the feet. Pay extra attention to your toes.

~ Keeping a thin, almost imperceptible, film of oil on the body is considered very beneficial for toning the skin and warming the muscles throughout the day. To conclude your massage, therefore, the oil should be rinsed off with mildly warm water and mild soap.

Mini-Massage (1–2 minutes)

~ If there is no time for a full-body massage, a short massage is still much better than none at all. The head and the feet are the most important parts of the body to cover, and this can be accomplished in a very short time. The mini-massage requires only about two tablespoons of oil.

~ Rub one tablespoon of warm oil into the scalp, using the small, circular motions described above. Using your palm, massage your forehead from side to side. Gently massage the temples, using circular motions, then gently rub the outside of the ears. Spend a few moments massaging the back and front of the neck.

~ With a second tablespoon of oil, massage both feet using the flat of the hand. Work the oil around the toes with your fingertips. Then vigorously massage the soles of the feet with brisk back-and-forth motions of the palms. Sit quietly for a few seconds to relax and soak in the oil, then bathe as usual.

As you can see, massage doesn't have to be complicated or expensive. Add a self-massage to your daily routine as a sign of your love for yourself. Make Sunday morning your family massage time, applying oil to those hard-to-reach places on your spouse's and children's backs. Gently stroke each other's foreheads before sleep and you will see an improvement in everyone's quality of rest.

Ask a friend to accompany you to your chemotherapy treatments and perform a gentle foot massage while you are receiving your medication. Allow their love and caring to infuse your being and blend with the drugs, adding healing spirit to the biochemistry of your care. Allow yourself to touch and be touched and you will notice the life-supporting effects on your mental and physical health.

Healing Sights

And God said: "Let there be light."
And there was light.
And God saw the light, that it was good.
GENESIS 1:3–4

Sight extends our reach across the universe. We hear things from miles away, smell things from yards at a distance, feel things within a few feet of us, and taste that which is on the threshold of entering our body. But light-years into the past and across vast expanses of space, we are able to see things that we can never hope to embrace with our other senses. From tiny specialized skin cells evolved the incredibly sophisticated extensions of our brain known as eyes. The great American photographer Ansel Adams experienced a profound change in his work when he realized that he was not taking photographs of objects in his environment but, rather, was capturing light on his camera film. Our amazing visual system, capable of perceiving electromagnetic radiation between two hundred and seven hundred billionths of a meter, must be one of the most remarkable products of evolution. My adaptable, rubbery lens is capable of focusing a few inches in front of me one moment and to a galaxy at an inconceivable distance the next. The receptors at the back of the eyeball can discriminate as little as a photon of light and can distinguish hundreds of colors on a bright day. Our world is so rich with potential visual stimuli that we must continuously filter out the vast bulk of light waves bombarding our optical receptors so that we are not overwhelmed with the kaleidoscope of shapes and colors that surround us. Close your eyes now and envision the room around you for a few moments. Now open your eyes and see how much you missed. There is simply too much to grasp, and so we focus on the limited information we need and screen out the rest.

From the time we are infants, we are attracted by visual stimuli. Brightly colored dangling ornaments are placed in our cribs to occupy our attention. Moving carousels and bouncing balls initially fascinate us, but we quickly hunger for more complex movements, available only in rapid-fire cartoons or skits on *Sesame Street*. As adults, hundreds of us stare transfixed at images reflected off a white screen while the latest iteration of a love or adventure story mesmerizes us for two hours at a stretch. Like food, sound, and touch, we ingest the sights around us, metabolizing them to create the substance of our body, mind, and soul.

The quality of our visual food provides us with nourishment or toxicity. Media barons may hotly debate the ratings of films, but can any intelligent person seriously dispute that exposing children and adults to relentless violence on television and in the movies erodes our sensitivity to the living beings around us? Many studies have shown that children who witness cruelty in the media are much more prone to use violence when feeling frustrated. The prevalence of violent crime in our society reflects our tolerance for primitive solutions to conflict as portrayed every day in our media. Fast-food establishments have learned that human beings will eat nutritionally empty substances if they are generously seasoned with sufficient sweetness and salt. Similarly, our entertainment moguls have learned that our general population will still wolf down artistically empty productions if the show is amply seasoned with sex and violence. These visual equivalents to junk food may not offer much nourishment, but they are easy to swallow.

Healing Images

How can we use this information to enhance our healing forces? First, we need to grasp that the information that we see translates into the biochemistry of our nervous system and ultimately our entire physiology. We should therefore be as careful about what we bring into our mind-body network through our eyes as we are about what enters our system through our mouths. When considering entertainment, choose movies and television programs that are inspirational and uplifting. Enjoy shows that are elevating, not degrading, to the human spirit. Watch great epics, inspiring adventures, nature documentaries, and lighthearted comedies that leave you feeling positive and hopeful. Avoid visual input that is abusive and disheartening.

Get out into nature and allow your eyes to absorb the beauty of the environment. Take walks in parks and natural preserves where you can saturate your senses with the sights, sounds, and smells of living, growing plants and animals. Walk along nearby lakes, rivers, and streams and imbibe their purifying influences. Spend time in the evening gazing at the moon and peering into the depths of the universe.

Expose yourself to sights that remind you of times when you were carefree and in the moment. Go to a playground and observe young children playing tag. Take your pooch to a dog park and watch young pups romping with each other. Watch a basketball game or go to a baseball game and sit in the bleachers, enjoying the timeless pleasure of our national pastime. Take a trip to Disneyland or Magic Mountain, and even if you can't stomach the Cyclone, observe and listen to the expressions of delight exhibited by children of all ages. Go to your local zoo and watch the animals and the people watching the animals. Use your eyes to connect you with this magnificent world, consuming the waves of electromagnetism with gusto and appreciation.

Bring pictures, photographs, and paintings of joyful and meaningful images into your home. Surround yourself with the smiling faces of your children, grandchildren, and beloved family and friends. Pull out pictures of past holidays and vacations and allow yourself to reexperience the joys from your past. Plan a trip to one of your favorite spots and look enthusiastically at travel brochures describing the delights that await you. Bring pictures or icons of deities that nurture you into your home—paintings of Christ, statues of Buddha, carvings of Krishna. Surround yourself with religious symbols that remind you of your connection to a higher power—a Star of David, a Tibetan Buddhist Tonka, a cast crucifix. Use your imagination to create a healing visual environment, customized to your needs and beliefs.

Wisdom traditions around the world have used visual symbols to activate deeper levels of healing and understanding. Depictions of Christian religious events, illustrations of Tibetan Buddhist creation myths, and a vast array of geometric diagrams portraying the relationships between outer and inner realities captivate our attention, uplifting our hearts and minds. Carl Jung, the greatest psychologist of our time, was fascinated by the power of visual symbols. Jung held that the ultimate goal of human life was to create wholeness and believed that circular, concentric images known as *mandalas* were an expression of our effort to integrate our individuality and universality.[26] He encouraged his patients to draw mandalas that might arise in their dreams, using them as tools to explore deeper levels of awareness. The great anthropologist Mircea Eliade once wrote, "The man who understands a symbol not only 'opens himself' to the objective world, but at the same time succeeds in emerging from his personal situation and reaching a comprehension of the universal."[27]

In Vedic tradition, visual symbols known as *Yantras* have been used for thousands of years to quiet the mind, eliciting a restful alertness response. Composed of basic geometric shapes—circles, triangles, and squares—these primordial forms bring us into present-moment awareness, calming our mental turbulence. Yantras can be considered the visual equivalent to mantras. One of the most ancient patterns is known as the *Shri Yantra*, representing the forces of expansion and contraction, masculinity and femininity, material and spiritual in the universe.

Gaze at the Shri Yantra below, allowing the various shapes to emerge and recede in your awareness. Record this brief guided visualization and play it to yourself while looking at the symbol.

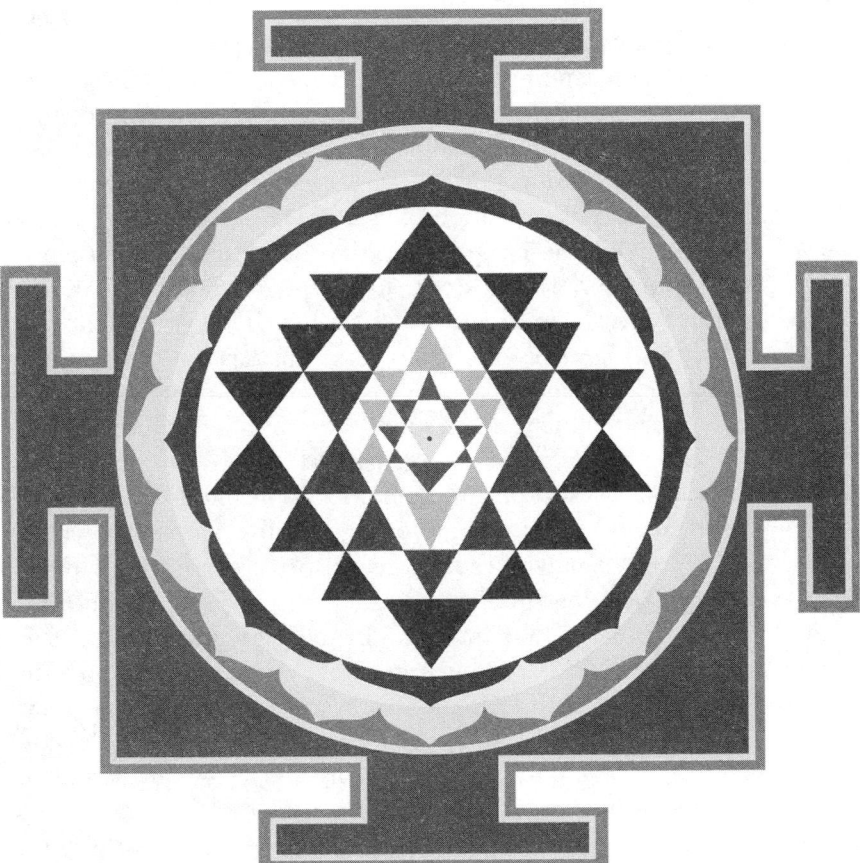

Figure 2 **Shri Yantra**

Yantra Meditation

~ As you look at the yantra, allow your eyes to focus on the center of it. This dot in the center is called the Bindu. The bindu represents the unity that underlies all the diversity of the physical world.

~ Now allow your eyes to see the triangle that encloses the center. The downward-pointing triangle represents the feminine creative power, while the upward-facing triangle represents male energy.

~ Allow your vision to expand to include the circles outside the triangles. They represent the cycles of cosmic rhythms. Within the image of the circle lies the notion that time has no beginning and no end. The farthest region of space and the innermost nucleus of an atom both pulsate with the same rhythmic energy of creation. It is all reflected right here. It is all reflected within you.

~ Notice the lotus petals outside the circle. Notice that they are pointing outward, as if opening. They illustrate the unfolding of our understanding. The lotus also represents the heart, the seat of the Self. When the heart opens, understanding comes.

~ The square at the outside of the yantra represents the world of form, the material world that our senses show us, the illusion of separateness, of well-defined edges and boundaries.

~ And finally at the periphery of the figure are four T-shaped portals, or gateways. Notice that they point toward the interior of the yantra, the inner spaces of life. They represent our earthly passage from the external and material to the internal and sacred.

~ Now take a moment to gaze into the yantra, letting the different shapes and patterns emerge naturally.

~ Allow your eyes to be soft, held loosely in focus. Your eyelids may droop a little. Perhaps your eyes will even seem to cross. Look at the center of the yantra on the screen. Now, without moving your eyes, gradually begin to expand your field of vision. Begin to include the edges of the page, expanding out to include the room. Continue expanding your field of vision until you are taking in information from greater than 180 degrees. Notice that all this information was already there all along— you just allowed it to enter your awareness. Now slowly reverse the process by refocusing back to the center of the yantra.

~ Now gently close your eyes. Allow the Shri Yantra to play on the screen of your inner vision for a minute before slowly opening your eyes.

Become friendly with a visual symbol that attracts you, and allow it to serve as a focal point for a visual meditation. Bring a symbol, painting, or photograph with you when you are undergoing treatment for your cancer and use it to calm your mind and empower you. There are many ways to enliven your healing response through the sense of sight. Just look around and you will see opportunities for enhancing your well being.

Healing Aromas

What's in a name?
That which we call a rose
By any other name would smell as sweet.
WILLIAM SHAKESPEARE

Virtue is like precious odors—
Most fragrant when they are incensed or crushed.
FRANCIS BACON

There was something about the home health nurse that disturbed Sylvia. Although she was consistently pleasant and professional, Sylvia found herself feeling literally sick to her stomach when the nurse paid a visit. After several appointments, it dawned on her that the cinnamon-based cologne the nurse wore was familiarly unpleasant. A similar heavy, sweet smell had been the signature fragrance of her music teacher with whom she had studied for many years. As a result of her tutelage, Sylvia became an accomplished pianist, but her teacher's harsh and critical style left its emotional marks.

Displaying uncommon directness, Sylvia told her story to the nurse, who took the information in a lighthearted manner, expressing her relief that there was not a more serious reason for Sylvia's obvious discomfort in her presence. From that point on, they developed a close friendship that endured throughout Sylvia's challenges with her ovarian cancer.

Our sense of smell is our most primitive sense. For most of our evolutionary journey we roamed the earth with our noses to the ground, inhaling the vapors of the environment. Until quite recently on the time scale of life, the bulk of the gray matter residing in our skulls was organized to process and respond to information entering through our noses. Data about sources of food, possible mates, potential competitors, and threatening predators could all be gathered through the olfactory system, enabling our prehuman ancestors to smell their way to choices that enhanced their chances for survival. As we expanded our capacity to remember and imagine through the development of layers of new nerve cells, our olfactory brain became buried, but continued to exert its primitive power on our interpretations and choices. Our sense of smell remains integral to our emotions and memories. As a medical student, I learned the functions of the smelling part of the brain through the mnemonic device of the "four F's"—feeding, fighting, fleeing, and the four-letter word for the action required to reproduce our species.

Our sense of smell links us with our deepest experiences. Imagine the aroma of the pine forest after a rain, the first wave of night-blooming jasmine, or a Thanksgiving turkey roasting in your grandmother's oven. Linked with each smell are multisensory memories—sights and sounds that remain hidden in our storehouse of impressions, seduced to the surface of our consciousness by the right fragrance. It may be decades since you last voluntarily inhaled the dried flower of the cannabis plant, but just a whiff of its acrid odor at a rock concert may conjure up a carnival of images and feelings from your past. Your mind may have buried the name and face of your high school sweetheart until years later when you pick up a blind date who happens to be wearing "her" signature cologne. The smell of a brand new car is so rich with positive associations that used-car salesmen spray synthetic air freshener in their "pre-owned" vehicles, hoping to evoke a similar level of enthusiasm. Likewise, real estate agents bake bread in the ovens of homes that have languished on the market, anticipating that a prospective buyer will be unable to resist the aroma of a "real" home.

Although augmenting the olfactory environment to intensify the healing process has been a component of therapeutic rituals for thousands of years, Western medicine is just beginning to recognize the value of aromatherapy. Since the dawn of time, medicine men and women around the globe have used incense from aromatic herbs and spices to create a sacred space while eliciting the healing response. As science seriously begins to explore the therapeutic effects of inhaling natural aromas, we are beginning to see validation of this ancient healing art.

How do we smell something? Molecules from a honeysuckle flower or freshly prepared minestrone soup are released into the air, where they are inhaled through the nose. These tiny messengers of matter dissolve in the linings of our nasal membranes, where they alter the chemistry of our very delicate olfactory nerves. These nerve cells communicate the smells of the world directly to our brains, where we decipher their codes and respond with attraction or repulsion. It has been estimated that human beings are capable of distinguishing ten thousand different smells, but we cannot come close to competing with some of our canine friends, who can detect one particle of a test aroma in ten trillion molecules of normal air.

Although we are only sniffing the surface of understanding as to how living beings can precisely discriminate aromas, headway is being made. The shape of a molecule seems to be critical in our ability to perceive its distinctive aroma. We can characterize seven primary olfactory codes from which the thousands of complex smells we distinguish are composed: floral, mint, musky, camphoric, pungent, ethereal, and putrid. The receptors in our olfactory nerves are triggered when one or more of these smelly chemicals penetrates the layers protecting them. Smell molecules may register for some time at a lower level of our consciousness before we become aware of them, as anyone who has burnt toast while engaged in a phone conversation can attest. We are receiving continuous information about the world through our snouts, which influences our thoughts, emotions, and behavior in subtle and not-so-subtle ways.

Aromatherapy has been used to reduce distress in patients undergoing medical procedures[28] and to encourage weight loss in people trying to shed their extra pounds.[29] A recent report from Japan tested the effects of aromatherapy on people admitted to a psychiatric hospital with depression and found that those who were exposed to a pleasant citrus fragrance had improvements in their moods, lower stress hormone levels, and better immune function and were able to be discharged on lower dosages of antidepressant medicines.[30]

Essential oils, derived from flowers, herbs, and spices, have effects that can be documented even in animals. A wide variety of different fragrances will have either relaxing or exciting influences on mice. In one study, citronella, lavender, lime, neroli, and sandalwood produced the most calming effect, while orange derivatives and thymol had the most activating influence.[31] The essential oils were concentrated in the bloodstream of the mice, demonstrating that what we inhale clearly enters our circulation. Other studies in animals show that if you couple a fragrance with a specific circumstance, exposure to the aroma will lead to a recall of the experience. For example, stressed mice will show elevations in fear hormones and impairment in their immune function. If they are allowed to relax in a safe cage that is filled with cedar wood shavings, the next time they are stressed, the harmful effects of the challenge can be offset by surrounding them with the smell of cedar.[32] The memory of a safe environment will be triggered by a pleasant smell. This process is known as neuroassociative conditioning.

Using Fragrance to Face Cancer

How can we make practical use of this information on aromatherapy to improve our well being if we are facing cancer? There are several ways we use the sense of smell at the Chopra Center to enhance a healing response. First, we can pay attention to the specific therapeutic effects of different aromas. As a general principle, the benefit of an essential oil will reflect the medicinal quality of the herb from which it came. Lavender has traditionally been used to calm an agitated mind, and the fragrance of this flowering herb has a tranquilizing effect. Black pepper is a digestive stimulant, as is its essential oil. Fennel seeds are useful to reduce acid indigestion, and the volatile oil derived from it can help to cool an irritated stomach. Other fragrant essential oils and their potential therapeutic benefits are listed below.

Essential oil	Latin name	Therapeutic effect	Indications
Camphor	*Cinnamomum camphora*	Decongestant, antiseptic, expectorant	Sinus congestion, bronchitis, allergies
Chamomile	*Anthemis nobilis*	Anti-inflammatory, antispasmodic, calming	Headaches, indigestion, insomnia
Eucalyptus	*Eucalyptus globulus*	Decongestant, antiseptic, expectorant	Sinus congestion, bronchitis, fatigue
Jasmine	*Jasmimum grandiflorum*	Detoxifying, calming, antidepressant	Depression, infection, inflammation
Peppermint	*Mentah piperita*	Analgesic, antiseptic, anti-inflammatory	Colds, indigestion, headache
Sandalwood	*Santalum album*	Calming, antipyretic, antiseptic	Insomnia, anxiety, inflammations

Mind-Body Principles and Aromas

As discussed in chapter 3, according to Ayurveda we can characterize our basic mind-body physiology in terms of three basic principles—movement, or "wind"; metabolism, or "fire"; and structure, or "earth." Just as we can

Balancing Wind, Fire, and Earth with Aromas

To Balance:	Wind	Fire	Earth
With symptoms of:	Anxiety, insomnia, weak appetite, constipation	Anger, irritability, hot flashes, diarrhea, inflammation	Weight gain, fluid retention, sinus congestion, lethargy
Use:	Vanilla, rose, cinnamon, ginger, basil, sandalwood, orange	Mint, lavender, chamomile, rose, sandalwood, jasmine, fennel, ylang-ylang	Cloves, ginger, basil, lime, thyme, basil, camphor, eucalyptus

use food to balance excesses in these principles, we can use the essential oils of herbs, spices, and flowers. If you are experiencing symptoms of a "wind" aggravation with anxiety, insomnia, fatigue, pain, and constipation, favor fragrances that are warm, sweet, and heavy. Commonly available aromas to ground the system include vanilla, sandalwood, rose, ginger, and patchouli. If you are experiencing imbalances in the "fire" element, with irritability, heartburn, fever, skin rashes, and diarrhea, use aromas that are cooling to the system, such as jasmine, sandalwood, lavender, clary sage, and mint. If you are feeling heavy, congested, lethargic, and retaining fluid, reflecting an aggravation of the "earth" principle, favor aromas that are light and spicy, such as juniper, orange, ginger, cinnamon, eucalyptus, and basil.

There are several ways to use aromas therapeutically. If the fragrance is in a volatile base, a few drops can be placed in a diffuser so that it permeates the air. There are several different types of diffusers, including those that apply heat to the essential oil and those that use a fan to carry the scent in a stream of air. If you are having trouble sleeping at night, diffuse some "wind"-pacifying aroma in your bedroom as you are getting ready for bed to help calm your agitated mind. If you are suffering with heartburn, diffuse a "fire"-pacifying fragrance in your dining room to cool your excessive digestive fire.

Aroma oils can also be applied to your skin, but they must be in a base oil that is meant for direct bodily contact. Otherwise, the essential oil can be quite irritating if placed directly on the skin. Place a few drops over your temples, on your upper lip beneath your nose, and over your neck. You will then carry the balancing fragrance with you wherever you go.

Neuroassociative Conditioning

We record each of our experiences through the sensory impressions that comprise it. Traces of sounds, sensations, sights, smells, and flavors are etched into our awareness by way of the neural networks in our brain. When we remember our wedding day, the birth of a child, or the death of a parent, we summon the recorded impressions, reconstructing the experience in our consciousness. Any one of the five senses may be predominant in our memory. In the examples above, it might be the music played during the wedding dance, the sight of our baby emerging from the birth canal, or the cold sensation when we touched our beloved mother's hand for the last time. Years later, we may hear the wedding song and be flooded with images and emotions as powerful as the originals.

We can use this understanding to associate powerful sensations with desirable experiences. The sense of smell is particularly useful in this process, for it is easy to couple an aroma to a comfortable and nourishing experience. Choose a distinctive fragrance that is attractive to you and diffuse it while you are meditating, listening to soothing, uplifting music, or receiving a massage. Create this association over several occasions so the aroma is intimately linked in your awareness with a pleasing, comfortable state. Then use the aroma when you need to invoke the serenity that you have connected with the fragrance. I have found this to be particularly useful when people are undergoing cancer treatments. By associating soothing music and a pleasant aroma with the tranquility of meditation, you can use the music and aroma while you are receiving chemotherapy to keep you open and centered. The anxiety and apprehension usually linked with medical procedures can often be substantially lessened through the use of positive, healing sensory associations.

Sensory Nourishment

We are not only what we eat, we are what we ingest, digest, and absorb though each of our five senses. When we are facing a serious illness, it is essential that we use our senses to bring only nourishing impulses into our physiology. Uplifting, inspiring sounds, loving, nurturing touch, beautiful, natural sights, and pleasing, delightful smells are the substrates that, combined with delectable food, create the essence of our minds and our bodies. The challenge of cancer requires that we make every choice as conscious as possible, asking the simple question: Will this increase or diminish my level of joy and well being? I encourage you to honor your body, mind, and spirit by allowing only the most life-supporting experiences to enter your life.

Commitment to Wholeness

Our bodies are the end products of our experiences and interpretations. To change our bodies, we need to change our experiences. Make a commitment to change your life in the direction of greater love and caring for yourself and those close to you.

1. I commit to creating a nurturing environment by choosing to surround myself with nourishing sounds, sensations, sights, tastes, and smells.

2. I will associate pleasing sounds and smells with a safe and comfortable state, using these sensory experiences to anchor my awareness when I am facing a challenging situation.

3. I will pay attention to subtle feelings of comfort and discomfort in my mind and my body and see whether they are reflecting toxic inputs from my environment. If there are sounds, sensations, sights, or smells that I can improve, I will do so.

CHAPTER 9

A Time to Every Purpose

Harmonizing with the Rhythms of Nature

And he shall be like a tree planted by the rivers of water, That bringeth forth his fruit in his season.—PSALMS 1:3

Rhythm is one of the principal translators between dream and reality. —DAME EDITH SITWELL

Harold was struggling to regain his sense of balance. He was undergoing chemotherapy treatments for his colon cancer, and although he seemed to be tolerating the drugs, he could not establish a comfortable daily routine. Despite feeling very fatigued, he was unable to fall asleep before one in the morning and usually awoke by six, tired and anxious. His appetite was suppressed and there was no regularity to his mealtimes. His moods fluctuated widely during the day, alternating between deep sadness and intense irritability. Although his large intestines had been reconnected after removal of the cancer, his bowel function was irregular and unpredictable.

When Harold came to see me, we agreed to focus on creating a daily routine that would enable him to regain a sense of rhythm in his life. He made every effort to get to sleep earlier, added a morning and evening meditation to his schedule, ate his main meal at lunch, and began walking for thirty minutes after dinner. Within a month his depression lifted, his energy level improved, and even his bowel habits showed some stability. His family reported that he was better-natured and easier to live with than he had been prior to his illness.

Life moves in eternal cycles of rest and activity. When physicists describe the subatomic world as having wavelike properties, they are acknowledging the primordial rhythms of the universe. What is a wave but the expression of energy alternating between its dynamic and quiet disguises? Everything that ever was, is, or will be has a beginning, middle, and end, arising from, and returning to, the eternal field of pure potentiality in an unending pulse of creation and dissolution.

Human beings are the most sophisticated product of nature's biological intelligence, and as expressions of nature, we are governed by seasons, cycles, and rhythms. From the vibration of elementary particles to the dance of galaxies, the throb of the universe can be perceived wherever we place our attention. Throughout our evolution, we have been moving to the beat of the cosmic drummer. Almost every plant and animal on this planet has developed in synchrony with the cycles on earth: the twenty-four-hour circadian rhythm of the earth spinning on its axis; the month-long lunar cycle, reflecting the moon's orbit around our watery planet; the twice daily tidal rhythms that dominated our evolution as we emerged from the ocean to land; and the annual cycle resulting from the 550-million-mile round-trip of the earth around our sun. The cycles of nature are hardwired into our nervous systems and influence our mental, emotional, and physical well being in both subtle and obvious ways.

I have defined health as the harmonious integration of environment, body, mind, and spirit. And what is the body but the perpetual recycling of the earth, water, and air that we exchange with the universe around us? From the time we were one-celled organisms to the development of the trillion cells that comprise our fully grown human bodies, our biological functions ebb and flow with the tides of nature. Every cell and tissue in our body expresses a rhythm, with times of vigorous activity and times of quietude. When our internal rhythms are in tune with the rhythms of nature, we experience vitality and joy. When we are out of sync with our environment, we notice dis-ease in body and mind.

A branch of science known as chronobiology has arisen over the past fifty years, dedicated to exploring the natural biological rhythms of life. Which cells, tissues, and systems in our body demonstrate rhythms and cycles? The answer is simple: every single biological expression—from the replication of DNA in a cell's nucleus to the secretion of hormones by our endocrine glands to our regulation of body temperature to the flow of air in our lungs—follows predictable cycles of rest and activity. If it is a feature of life, it is dancing in rhythm with nature.

Cancer cells, however, lose much of their natural rhythmicity.[1] Unlike normal cells that take time for some cellular rest and rejuvenation, cancer cells compulsively march on, ignoring advice to stop and smell the roses. In prior chapters, I've discussed how we can view malignancy as loss of the memory of wholeness. What is it that generates a sense of unity among parts? In the same way that musicians align themselves with their orchestra through rhythm, the concert of our mind-body symphony depends upon each cell's playing its part on time. The timing of physiological processes is key to good health. When a cell or tissue loses the beat, it fails to contribute to wholeness. Our goal, then, when facing illness, is to enliven harmony and rhythm in every phase of our lives.

The Rhythms of Nature

Long before primitive life forms emerged in our primordial oceans, the earth was turning on its axis, generating day and night. As biological beings developed, this circadian ("circa" = around, "dia" = day) rhythm encouraged cyclical patterns of rest and activity in cells and organisms. Hundreds of millions of years later, we can detect these daily rhythms throughout our bodies. Our reproduction of genetic material and our manufacture of essential proteins show highs and lows within a twenty-four-hour cycle.[2] Our heart rate, blood pressure, breathing pattern, and body temperature all cycle predictably throughout the day. The basic behaviors we take for granted—sleeping, eating, and drinking—are paced by very basic rhythm generators in our nervous system. Almost every hormone in our endocrine system follows a diurnal pattern with phases of activity and quiescence. Acid secretion in the stomach, detoxifying enzymes in the liver, absorption and release of salts in the kidneys, and the aggressiveness of immune cells all ride a daily wave with peaks and troughs of activity.

How can we use this information to improve our health? We need to recognize that until very recently, human beings stayed closely in tune with the rhythms of nature. Since pulling ourselves up on two legs, we arose with the sun, ate at midday, and retired when sunlight faded in the evening. But life for our species changed dramatically when Thomas Edison harnessed the power of electricity in the late nineteenth century, for since that time we have enjoyed the freedom to create day and night at will. If we so choose, we can now snack on a frozen pizza at midnight, watch television until three in the morning, and shop for toothpaste in a twenty-four-hour pharmacy at the crack of dawn. Although we all cherish the conveniences of modern technology, it has created the impression that we no longer need to pay attention to nature's rhythms. Yet we pay a price for ignoring nature's seasons. When we are out of sync with our environment, we experience fatigue, difficulty with sleeping, indigestion, and emotional turbulence.

It is not difficult to reestablish balance in our daily routines. It simply requires paying attention to clues from our inner and outer environments. I recommend trying the daily routine described below. Notice how it influences your quality of life.

Morning

- ~ Wake without an alarm clock by 7 A.M.
- ~ Brush your teeth and clean your tongue.
- ~ Drink a glass of warm water to encourage regular elimination.
- ~ Empty your bowels and bladder.
- ~ Massage your body with oil.
- ~ Bathe.
- ~ Perform light exercise.
- ~ Meditate.
- ~ Eat breakfast.
- ~ Take a midmorning walk.

Midday

- ~ Make lunch your main meal of the day.
- ~ Sit quietly for five minutes after eating.
- ~ Walk to aid digestion for five to fifteen minutes.
- ~ Meditate in the late afternoon.

Evening

- ~ Eat a light to moderate dinner between five and seven o'clock.
- ~ Sit quietly for five minutes after eating.
- ~ Walk to aid digestion for five to fifteen minutes.

Bedtime

~ Perform light activity in the evening.
~ Go to bed early, but at least three hours after dinner.
~ Do not read, eat, or watch TV in bed

It's best to awaken without an alarm clock at about 6 A.M. If you cannot imagine rising this early, try leaving an east- or south-facing window uncovered so that the rising sun will arouse you. I don't recommend alarm clocks because they all tend to be so jarring, making your very first morning experience one of stress. There are people whose circadian rhythms have become so out of line that they find it extremely difficult to get into this pattern. If you are having trouble sleeping at night or if you've never paid much attention to lifestyle regularity, I recommend that you use an alarm clock and wake up very early (before 5 A.M.) every morning for several days in a row. If you avoid napping during the day, you will soon be drifting off to sleep by ten in the evening and this will reset your whole cycle.

Brush your teeth, gently cleaning your tongue if it is coated. It is common while undergoing chemotherapy to have a foul or sour taste in the mouth, particularly when you first arise. According to Ayurveda, this reflects your body's level of toxicity and is a sign to pay extra attention to, allowing only nourishing food and sensory impressions into your system. It is helpful to drink plenty of warm water throughout the day, beginning after you clean your mouth. Drinking some hot water or herbal tea stimulates peristaltic motion so that you will be able to effortlessly empty your bowels and bladder.

Perform a daily oil massage before your bath or shower, which benefits your skin and general health. I also suggest a light set of yoga postures or stretching, followed by twenty to thirty minutes of meditation. Then eat breakfast if you are hungry and take a short walk after your meal if time allows.

Although few of us follow this advice, most people feel better if they eat their largest meal at noontime. This was the natural practice in most societies until the Industrial Revolution, when it became inconvenient for employees to take the time off from work to eat a large midday lunch. A balanced, well-cooked meal at noon can have a beneficial effect on your entire daily routine. Sit for a few minutes after lunch and take a short walk if possible.

Perform your second meditation in the late afternoon or in the early evening before dinner. This facilitates the release of accumulated stress from the day and prepares you for your evening activities. Eat a lighter dinner around six o'clock, and then sit quietly for five minutes after eating. An evening walk after your meal will aid digestion and is a great time to connect with your family.

Getting Rest

Although some people find themselves sleeping more under stress, most people facing a serious illness find that their sleep is disturbed. As a general rule, we use activity to release internal pressures. At the end of a day, when it is time to turn things off, an agitated mind may not be so willing to disengage, even though the body is calling for much-needed rest. Lack of rejuvenating sleep compounds the problem as a person worries about how he or she will be able to function the next day without adequate rest.

There are some simple maneuvers that I have found helpful for people who suffer from occasional insomnia. Like getting an infant to sleep through the night, a regular routine is invaluable in conditioning the mind to shift gears. If you are having trouble sleeping, start by limiting your activity after dinner. Have the intention of slowing down in preparation for bed. Avoid vigorous exercise, violent television shows, and intensive mental work whenever possible. If you have been focusing intensely and your mind is very active right before bedtime, it will take you longer to fall asleep. Try being in bed with the lights off by ten o'clock and certainly no later than eleven. The following ritual often proves helpful in getting to sleep:

~ An hour before bedtime, put on some calming, soothing music.
~ Diffuse a relaxing fragrance of essential aroma oil such as lavender, vanilla, chamomile, or vetiver in your bedroom. Use this aroma only at bedtime.
~ Prepare a hot bath and put a few drops of the same essential aroma oil you are diffusing into the bath water.
~ Perform a ten-minute massage with almond or sesame oil.
~ Turn down the lights and take a leisurely bath.
~ After your bath, drink a cup of hot milk with nutmeg and cardamom or a cup of hot chamomile or valerian tea.
~ Go directly to bed, allowing your attention to be on your breath as you fall asleep.
~ If you have a sleeping partner, encourage him or her to follow the same routine so you are not disturbed just as you are falling asleep.

~   Try using a soothing heating pad or warm water bottle on your abdomen as you are lying in bed. Be certain that they are warm and not hot so you don't burn yourself as you are dozing off.
~   Do not read, talk on the phone, eat, or watch television in bed.

Sound sleep is a key component of good health. Studies have shown that even a few hours of sleep deprivation can diminish immune function until the sleep debt is repaid.[3] Our quality of rest is best before midnight, so that eight hours of sleep between 10 P.M. and 6 A.M. will provide deeper rejuvenation than eight hours between 1 A.M. and 9 A.M. If you have always considered yourself a "night person," try gradually getting to bed earlier until you are in the habit of being asleep by eleven. There are people who have a lifelong pattern of staying up later and sleeping later in the morning, but studies have shown that those who maintain this routine are more likely to have periods of sadness, fatigue, and anxiety.[4] Although it may seem like a minor issue when you are facing a serious illness, establishing a healthy daily routine can make a substantial impact on your well being.

Seasonal Cycles

We've all noticed the effect of the seasons on our mental and physical health. Few of us fail to experience some change in our mood as the days get shorter approaching the winter solstice, or the uplifting influence of spring as the earth awakens from her cold slumber. Over millions of years of evolutionary time, we developed and adapted to the changing seasons by internalizing the rhythms of nature. Because the earth is tilted on its axis, the outside temperature and the hours of natural light rise and fall throughout the year. These perpetual oscillations influence many levels of our lives. The release of mood-regulating chemicals, our attraction to the opposite sex, and the timing of societal celebrations all dance to the tempo of the seasonal percussionist.

In human beings, as in most animals, melatonin is the primary chemical messenger that attunes our inner clock with that of nature. This process of harmonizing our mind-body cycle with cycles in the environment is known as entrainment. Melatonin is produced by the pineal, a small gland near the center of the brain, which transforms light energy into biochemical messengers. The pineal gland continuously eavesdrops on the visual system, responding to the amount of light available in the world by releasing more or less melatonin. The varied effects of melatonin are fascinating. Fertility in cows, winter coat growth in foxes, and hibernation in bears are all influenced by this chemical.

Melatonin in humans has a major effect on our sleep/wake cycles, hormone secretion, mood, and immune function. Jet lag is a common problem related to melatonin that almost everyone has experienced, occurring most often when we travel across multiple time zones. Jet lag results from a lack of harmony between our internal clock and the messages our brain is receiving from the time-shifted environment in which we find ourselves. The quickest way to adapt to a new time zone is by immediately following the routine of the environment in which you've arrived. Eat your next meal at the appointed hour and get into bed at the time appropriate for the site you are visiting. Preliminary studies have suggested that a dose of melatonin (one milligram per time zone) several hours before bedtime can help reset the biological clock, but its most appropriate use and potential side effects are still to be defined.[5]

A recently recognized condition known as Seasonal Affective Disorder (SAD) describes the depression that many people experience during the short days of winter. In addition to mood changes, people with SAD often gain weight, crave calorie-rich foods, and feel sleepy during the day. This condition is related to alterations in melatonin production and can be improved by exposure to bright lights during the day.[6] It is particularly prevalent in northern regions, where winter hours of sunlight exposure are limited. Many people experience lesser manifestations of winter sadness, accounting in part for the popularity of southern resort spots during the winter months. Ancient solar baskers who often revered the sun as a god noticed the healing effect of the sun on our emotional states. People today who feel their winter depression lifting as the days lengthen would probably agree with our ancestral sun worshippers' view of our life-giving star.

How can we use this information about seasonal effects to improve our well being throughout the year? Although we can attempt to ignore or override nature's signals, the best approach is to listen and honor her messages. As the days become shorter, pay attention to the signals you are receiving from the environment, not from your timepiece. Get to bed earlier, awaken earlier, and adjust your meal and meditation times accordingly. Dress appropriately for the weather and choose foods that are balancing to the qualities being expressed in the environment. During the dry, cold, blustery autumn, choose "wind"-pacifying foods that are warmer and heavier like hearty soups, stews, and casseroles. During summer, when the "fire" element predominates, choose foods, clothing, and activities to keep you cool. During the wet, cold spring season, favor lighter, warmer foods and spices, and be certain to dress appropriately to stay warm and dry. Use all your senses to balance environmental influences, paying attention to the moods of nature, remembering that the nature of nature is cyclical change.

Seasons, Cycles, and Cancer

What is known about the relationship between cancer and our normal biological cycles? There is an explosive amount of information emerging that has the potential to dramatically alter the way we provide cancer treatment. A number of recently uncovered clues hint at the possibility that understanding the changes in rhythm in cancer can help us improve health. We have learned that certain cancers occur more commonly during some seasons than others. For example, breast cancer is more frequently diagnosed in the spring months, and prostate cancer is most commonly discovered in the winter. This suggests that our pineal glands may be the source of some natural cancer-fighting substance, which rises and falls throughout the year.[7] Whether this substance works through our immune systems or from a direct antitumor effect, we may uncover a new class of drugs based upon a natural medicine from our inner pharmacy.

Men and women with cancer commonly lose their usual cyclical hormonal patterns, reinforcing the concept that a fundamental feature of malignancy is the loss of physiological rhythm. We can take advantage of cancer's loss of natural rhythm by timing chemotherapy to capitalize on the differences between malignant and healthy cells. There are four important questions that need to be considered when developing *chronotherapy* (timed therapy) for cancer.

~ When are the cancer cells most sensitive to the chemotherapy drug?
~ When are the normal cells in the organ with cancer least sensitive to the drug?
~ When are our immune and blood-producing cells least vulnerable to the drug?
~ When are the organs that break down and eliminate the drug (liver and kidney) most active?

If we knew the answers to these questions, we could design a cancer treatment protocol that gave medicines when our normal cells were resting, the cancer cells were most active, and our elimination organs were relatively quiet. Then, any medicine administered would have maximal effect against cancer cells, cause minimal harm to our healthy cells, and could be given in the lowest possible dosage.

We are beginning to learn the answers to the above questions, although we still have a way to go. The toxicity of a cancer medicine is vastly different, depending upon when it is administered.[8] Mice are five times more likely to die from a nighttime dose of the chemotherapy drug arabinosyl cytosine (AraC) than if they receive the same exact dose during the day. People receiving floxuridine (FUDR) for colon cancer at six in the evening will have less nausea, diarrhea, and mouth soreness than if they are given the same total dosage evenly distributed throughout a twenty-four-hour period.

The efficacy of a chemotherapy drug in treating a cancer may be greater when given at one time of the day versus another.[9] For example, children with leukemia have better outcomes if they receive their maintenance dosage of chemotherapy in the evening rather than in the morning. Some of the improvement results from their greater tolerance to higher doses of the medications that have less toxicity when given at certain times of the day.

Although progress is being made in applying our expanding knowledge of biological rhythms to cancer therapy, we are learning that not everyone and not every cancer responds in the same way. Scientists are trying to find simple ways of determining when a person's normal cells are resting and when the cancer cells are most active. These chemical flags of cellular activity are sometimes called "chronomes" and include substances such as carcinoembryonic antigen (CEA) and alpha-fetoprotein (AFP). The hope is that we will soon be capable of using simple tests to determine the best time to administer cancer medicines in order to create maximal benefit with minimal side effects.

I recommend discussing the issue of chronotherapy with your doctor. Although this field is in its infancy, there is a growing body of information that may help guide the optimal timing of your treatments. Programmable automatic drug-delivery devices are now available to administer medications at set times, allowing for customized schedules to be developed.

The Rhythm of Life

I sometimes fantasize about simpler times, when the world moved more slowly. It took longer to get from one place to another, so we were forced to focus on the journey as much as the destination. We were more in tune with our environment because we had to pay closer attention for our survival and well being. Nature was revered and respected for her power. If we wanted to participate in the cosmic dance, it was clear that she was leading and we were following. We learned that the more we honored the rhythms of the world, the better we felt and the more likely we were to fulfill our physical, emotional, and spiritual needs.

Nature, however, is not always so gentle. As human beings we are impelled to develop increasingly sophisticated technologies that insulate ourselves from her impetuous moods. We began with fire, shelters, and the skins of animals, graduating over time to indoor heating, condominiums, and down parkas. In our desperate need for uninterrupted information, we developed fax machines, cable television, and voice mail. We hoped to save time but discovered that we had more bits of data to contend with than ever before. Just consider how you would feel if you still had to use a rotary telephone to make your calls!

It's time for us as individuals and communities to reconnect with the rhythms of life that pulse through every star in our cosmos and every cell in our bodies. A serious illness is a call from our soul to reorder our priorities and search for the balance that is our true nature. Harmonize with nature's songs, synchronize with nature's rhythms—they are calling you to wholeness.

Commitment to Wholeness

Our bodies are the end products of our experiences and interpretations. To change our bodies, we need to change our experiences. Make a commitment to change your life in the direction of greater love and caring for yourself and those close to you.

1. I commit to establishing a daily routine in tune with the rhythms of nature.

2. I will focus attention on the seasonal variations, choosing behaviors balancing to the cyclical changes in my environment.

3. If I am having difficulty sleeping, I will work on establishing a regular sleep routine that is pacifying to all five senses.

CHAPTER 10

Emotional Healing

Riding the Turbulent Wave of Feelings

Emotion is the chief source of all becoming conscious. There can be no transforming of darkness into light and of apathy into movement without emotion.—CARL JUNG

> To a student whose heart is full of love,
> Who has seen beyond his senses and passions,
> The teacher will reveal the Lord of Love.
> —MUNDAKA UPANISHAD

Laura was the caregiver in the family. Not only did she provide primary emotional support for her husband and three children, she was also the backbone of her birth family, relied upon heavily by her two younger sisters. After her father's death, she assumed the added responsibility for her mother's well being, making herself available to lend a hand whenever needed.

When she learned that the lump in her breast was cancerous, Laura was overwhelmed by powerful emotions. Adept at giving to others, she was extremely uncomfortable asking help for herself. And her family that so depended upon her for their needs had difficulty providing her with the support she needed. An unprecedented sense of despair and hopelessness overpowered her.

After trying but receiving little benefit from an antidepressant medicine, Laura joined a cancer support group. Here she learned that it was acceptable to express her needs and feelings and found people who could embrace and nurture her. She

153

gained insight into her unhealthy pattern of giving to others at the expense of exhausting herself. As she successfully navigated her way through her cancer treatments, she also discovered aspects of herself that had been dormant since childhood. Her depression gradually lifted, and she was able to establish more balanced relationships with her beloved family.

Our emotions are a fathomless ocean of thoughts and feelings. On any given day our emotional sea may be calm with clear visibility or intensely turbulent, generating a fear of drowning in the overpowering waves. Emotions express themselves through our flesh and bones, demanding our attention and refusing to be rational. We call them feelings because we feel them in our body—a tightness in our gut, a pressure in our heart, a strangling sensation in our throat. I can read about a political development in Iraq, feeling relatively little, and then move to the sports page, where I may get emotionally charged upon learning that my favorite basketball team lost in the final seconds of a game. A thought without a corresponding physical sensation is just an idea, but when it affects me at a visceral level it becomes an emotion. The wisdom of the body is expressed through our experience of comfort or distress, and our feelings are the distilled essence of our mental and physical states. We meet a friend and ask, "How are you feeling?" seeking to palpate her emotional pulse. She responds with her current mark on the emotional gauge—"fine," "fabulous," or "miserable"—providing a snapshot of her current state of well being. Although we take our feelings to be the measure of reality, at a deeper level we know that reality could not possibly change as quickly as our emotional states.

It may sound paradoxical, but when you have a serious illness such as cancer, your initial psychological distress is healthy. The anxiety and sadness that you feel is a natural response to your perception of loss. The physical sensations that arise serve to capture your attention and mobilize your inner healing resources. Your discomfort is the fire alarm alerting you that urgent intervention is necessary. The challenge we face when confronting a serious threat is how to use our feelings to grow, learn, and expand our repertoire of responses.

The Emotions of Cancer

There is no question that having cancer generates a storm of emotions. We would not be human if we did not have strong feelings as a consequence of learning about a serious illness. But a question that has been raised for hundreds of years is whether certain emotional styles can *create* cancer. Over the years, psychologists have suggested that people who have difficulty expressing strong feelings and who feel they have little control over their lives are more likely to develop cancer than people who are comfortable expressing their feelings and feel empowered in their lives.[1] For the past thirty years, it has been suggested that there are "cancer-prone" personality characteristics, but there remains considerable controversy as to how meaningful these traits are. Do people who keep their feelings to themselves send less healthy messages to their immune cells? Or does facing cancer cause people to become more withdrawn and less expressive of their emotions? Despite many studies focusing on this issue, the jury is still out.[2] As discussed in earlier chapters, we know that our state of mind directly and rapidly influences our ability to identify and respond to potentially harmful influences. But are there better and worse ways to handle stress? And more important, can we change our emotional responses to life's challenges?

If you are currently facing cancer, you may be asking, "What is the value of learning now about possible personality traits that may have contributed to my risk?" Certainly, there is no benefit in blaming yourself for qualities that you may have acquired in early childhood and no value in reproaching yourself for choices you could have made in the past. The usefulness of looking at these characteristics is in considering whether it's possible to develop a healthier emotional style now. What's the point in changing now if you already have cancer? The answer I offer is that a healthier emotional life is its own reward.

I have suggested earlier that cancer provides an opportunity to recreate your life in a globally healthier way. A critical component of health includes taking responsibility for your feelings. Responsibility means the ability to have a creative response. It is altogether different from blame. I suggested in chapter 1 that cancer compels us to ask ourselves important questions. Two that are relevant here are: "What is the deeper significance of this illness?" and "What is cancer telling me about the way I am living my life?" If we are prepared to honestly address these questions, profound transformation and healing can occur.

If you are willing to explore this issue further, look at some of the personality traits that *may* be more prevalent in people at risk for developing cancer and see how many apply to you.[3] Are you:

~ Overly cooperative
~ Appeasing
~ Unassertive
~ Overly patient

~   Conflict-averse
~   Compliant
~   Uncomfortable expressing anger or strong emotions

None of these traits is inherently undesirable or inappropriate. In fact, if we looked at people at risk for heart disease they would have almost the opposite personality traits—being uncooperative, demanding, impatient, conflict-oriented, and willing to express anger without concern for its impact on others. The issue, then, is not one of right and wrong, but rather of balance.

We've explored the fight-or-flight response as our most primitive way of coping with a threatening environment. When your life is in jeopardy, you are neurologically wired to react vigorously by running away or engaging in conflict. Since in modern life neither of these two options is rarely adaptive or acceptable, we have developed slightly more sophisticated approaches, known as psychological defense mechanisms. These are the various coping mechanisms that provide us some sense of control over our lives. Because most of us feel distress when we are out of control, these coping strategies may be thought of as control strategies, or when they are less adaptive, control dramas, designed to lessen psychological distress. Rather than physically fighting when we are feeling threatened or challenged, we may become sarcastic, intimidating, or verbally abusive. Instead of physically running away, we may choose to withdraw, become uncommunicative, and shut down emotionally. We developed our repertoire of control strategies in childhood when we were learning and adapting to the emotional styles of our primary family members and caregivers. We may have learned early in our development that an aggressive style was necessary in order for our needs to be met. Alternatively, we may have received the message that expressing strong emotions was never acceptable.

If you are a person who has difficulty expressing your feelings, ask yourself the questions listed below. I have found it most useful to either answer these questions aloud or write your answers in a journal. By aloud I mean talking to yourself in a place where you won't be disturbed, or communicating with a friend or counselor who is willing and able to accept the range of your emotions. Although you may feel uncomfortable at first speaking audibly when no one else is around, I have found it more useful than simply thinking about your answers. You will probably find yourself having a conversation with an imaginary person who is an amalgamation of the voices of resistance or judgment you are carrying in your heart and mind.

1. Is it true that I have been reluctant or unable to openly express my feelings?
2. Do I believe that I deserve to express my feelings to my family and friends?
3. What do I believe are the consequences of expressing my feelings?
4. What am I afraid will happen if I begin to express my feelings now?

If you believe that it's desirable for you to be more open with your emotions, allow the changes to unfold naturally. Practice expressing yourself in a manner that does not engender resistance. The most common self-limitation that people encounter in their emotional lives is the tendency to blame others for how they are feeling. The most empowering insight that engenders true emotional freedom is the realization that each of us is responsible for our own feelings. A person, situation, or circumstance may trigger an emotional response in us, but no one and nothing can make us feel a certain way without our implicit permission. Someone can be intimidating or demoralizing, but it is our choice whether to be intimidated or demoralized. Most of us are so accustomed to saying things like "You hurt my feelings!" or "You make me so angry!" that the concept that we actually have a choice as to how to react may seem ludicrous. Yet we have all had the experience of being able to laugh off a caustic comment from someone for whom we have limited regard, but feeling deeply wounded by a subtle suggestion of disappointment expressed by someone whose approval we crave. It's clearly our interpretation of the experience that determines our emotional response to it.

Everyone dealing with cancer experiences distress, because serious illness always activates our deepest fears of loss. Loss of energy, comfort, time, independence, and control are all naturally accompanied by sadness, but not necessarily by despair or hopelessness. It is often the minor disappointments that compound our distress—an insensitive comment from a health care provider, lack of compassionate support from a spouse, or an unkind remark by a friend. It is in the context of these lesser challenges that we often have the opportunity to gain insight into ourselves, acquiring wisdom and awareness in the process.

Processing Emotional Upsets

The processing of emotions requires paying attention to both our minds and our bodies. This means listening to the message that the feeling is carrying, and acknowledging the sensations in our body. Learning to communicate directly with the people we love reduces stress and frees up our life energy. Emotions that we accept without judgment provide an opportunity for personal growth and self-reflection that can be empowering to our family and ourselves. When facing a challenging circumstance, the following process can be helpful in moving through the emotional upsets that create needless additional stress.

1. *Identify* the emotion you are feeling: "I feel _____." It may be angry, sad, hurt, betrayed, abandoned, rejected, frustrated, or hopeless. As clearly as possible, define and describe what you are feeling. Putting a label on your feelings helps to focus your attention and establish some limits for the emotions that may at first feel overwhelming. It is the first step in channeling the powerful energy of the feeling in an evolutionary direction.

2. *Observe* the feelings in your body. An emotion is a thought associated with physical sensations. Our thoughts trigger bodily reactions, which have a chemistry of their own. The physiological expressions of stress cannot be instantaneously shut off. Rather, the frothy energy of the emotion must be dissipated before the emotion can be processed further. Having identified what it is you are feeling, simply allow yourself to feel the emotions. Consciously direct your breath to the location in your body that is holding the pressure and allow each exhalation to release some of the tension. Embrace the sensation in your body with your attention and have the intention to release the emotional charge, recognizing that these are your feelings, but they are not you. By allowing yourself to experience the physical sensations, some of the emotional energy will dissipate and you'll be able to hear the message the emotion is carrying.

3. *Express* the emotion, in private, to yourself. You can write about your feelings or speak them out loud. I have found that keeping a journal just for this purpose is invaluable. Write freely and without judgment about whatever thoughts are racing through your mind. Resist the impulse to filter, and don't worry if you are writing things you would never feel comfortable saying aloud. Often when journaling, distant memories of similar situations may surface. Take advantage of the access that your current upset is providing to past emotional traumas and write about them, too. Use language that boldly and honestly conveys what you are feeling. Allow yourself to express all that you need to about the situation.

I am convinced of the therapeutic benefit of journaling. The very process of expressing our feelings in writing helps us to gain a perspective on them. When I journal, I often find that I start laughing at myself as I document my self-righteous indignation at a perceived injustice. The benefits of journaling have even been scientifically studied. College students who write about upsetting events show improvement in their immune function and make fewer visits to the campus health clinic.[4] A recent study from the University of Auckland Medical School in New Zealand demonstrated that medical students who wrote about traumatic events in their lives generated more antibodies in response to a vaccination.[5] It has been consistently shown that the more a person is willing to express their strong negative feelings in writing, the more their immune status and overall health improve. Writing about the stressful events in our lives may be one of the healthiest ways available to us to process and discharge our strong feelings.

4. *Release* the emotion through some ritual. If you have expressed your feeling, the turbulence in your mind will have calmed, but your body still needs to release the pressure that has been raised. Some form of physical activity is usually best for this. Go for a walk, dance, swim, perform yoga, or do breathing exercises—anything that will help you to discharge the emotion from your physiology. If you are feeling angry, pound a pillow, throw rocks in the ocean, or yell at God. Do something that gives your body a sense of relief, without causing any harm to your environment. Allow your body to detoxify and acknowledge the release of your feelings as you are doing the activity.

5. *Share* the emotion with someone who can listen attentively to you without trying to solve your problem. Conscious listening is a skill that takes practice. A valuable communication procedure shared with us by our friend Robert Gass makes use of a talking object. A talking object has been used by Native Americans to ritualize important communications for thousands of years. Identify a beautiful stone or small piece of polished wood as your object, which is used exclusively for meaningful communication sessions. Holding the object in your hands, express your feelings honestly, openly, and without blame. The person with whom you are communicating has the role of listening attentively without interruption, secure in the knowledge that he or she will have an opportunity to respond and be heard. Speak from your heart until you feel complete, remembering to take responsibility for your own feelings. Then transfer the talking object to your partner and provide him or her with the same attention you received while speaking. This procedure enhances communication and reduces the possibility of the discussion degenerating into an argument of blame.

As you are speaking, try to avoid expressions such as "You hurt my feelings!" or "You always make me feel this way!" Rather, use language that does not evoke defensiveness and resistance, such as "My feelings were hurt when you said . . ." When it is your turn to listen, be careful not to interrupt the other person in attempting to defend yourself. Simply listen attentively, receiving the messages that are useful and let those that are not of value pass by.

6. *Rejuvenate!* If you have moved through the five steps listed above, all the while being aware of your responsibility for your own feelings, you have accomplished something great. It takes conscious awareness and a commitment to personal growth to go through the process described above, so reward yourself for your good work. If both people in the relationship are committed to deepening their level of intimacy through conscious communication, there is no issue that cannot be handled in a loving and respectful manner. If you are lucky enough to be in such a relationship, celebrate each successful processing together. Do something nice for your partner and yourself. Give each other a massage, go to a movie, enjoy a delicious meal—be open to receiving nourishment.

Let's explore a situation that illustrates the possibility of transforming a potentially distressing interaction into a positive, life-affirming experience. You go to your oncologist for a three-month checkup after your chemotherapy course has been completed. During your exam, he casually mentions that a recent study showed that people who underwent your cancer treatment survived an average of three years, compared to less than eighteen months for those on an older treatment protocol. Although your doctor meant to reassure you with this information, you immediately feel panicked. Since you are now two years out from your diagnosis you start to worry that you have less than a year of life left. Arriving home, you begin the process of emotional clearing:

1. Identify: You identify the emotions you are facing as fear and anger. You fear physical discomfort and loss of quality time with your family. You are angry that your doctor gave you the information in a way you perceived as insensitive.

2. Observe: You practice meditation for a few minutes, directing your attention to your body. You become aware of a knot in your stomach and a sense of restriction in your chest. You allow the pressure in your body to release with each breath. As you do so, some of the panicky feelings begin to subside.

3. Express: You begin writing in your journal, describing your fears and sense of injustice that a good person such as yourself should have to

go through this process, while so many other people are healthy. As you express these thoughts, tears begin to flow and you feel some emotional release and relief. You then begin to have new thoughts in which you realize that your doctor was trying to provide you with encouragement, not a death sentence. You decide that you will discuss the situation directly with him that day.

4. Release: You go for a brisk walk, planning what you want to say to your doctor in a way that expresses your concerns without creating resistance. You feel empowered and confident that you can express your needs directly.

5. Share: You call your doctor that afternoon, asking if he has a few minutes to talk to you. He is available and listens as you express your concerns honestly and responsibly. He immediately apologizes for being insensitive to the effect his words had on you and explains that he told you the information to reassure you that his treatment recommendations were appropriate. He also tells you that people in the study who were disease-free for two years had an excellent chance of remaining healthy.

6. Rejuvenate: You feel much better and arrange to have a massage that evening. You call your sister, describing what you went through, and you make plans to go out to dinner at your favorite restaurant.

Some emotional upsets are best dealt with this way, but others may not be so easily released. When experiencing physical pain or an impending loss, expressing your distress will not magically cause the pain to vanish. Sometimes, when there is simply too much stress to deal with at once, psychological coping mechanisms that utilize denial or suppression of feelings may be most adaptive.[6] This is particularly true when people first learn that they have cancer and must consider a number of immediate decisions regarding diagnosis and treatment. At this time, considering the deeper psychological significance of the illness may be inappropriate and unhelpful. Other coping mechanisms such as using goal-oriented activity as a diversion (cleaning the house, organizing your files), consciously directing your attention away from anxiety-producing thoughts (using positive affirmations), and tackling problems head-on (surfing the Web to learn everything you can about cancer) may be effective ways to deal with a threatening situation. You will know when it is the right time to dive more deeply into the meaning of your illness and your emotional patterns. For every aspect of health, it's essential that we use the best tool for the task, and this certainly applies to our psychological strategies.

Weathering the Emotional Storms

I encourage my patients to use as many healing strategies as possible, recognizing that each of us has unique needs and responds in different ways to life's many offerings. When a person is forced to confront the fears that cancer engenders, the first goal is to reduce distress to a manageable level while striving to reestablish emotional equilibrium. Once some semblance of balance is present, the opportunity to dive more deeply into the emotional and spiritual meaning of the illness presents itself. At every stage, there are five components that I've found to be valued allies in the healing process:

1. Meditation, prayer, and visualization techniques
2. Emotional expression
3. Family support
4. Accurate information about the illness
5. Medical interventions

Each of these approaches addresses a different but important facet of the emotional needs of people facing cancer.

Meditation, Prayer, and Visualization Techniques

By now you know my belief that taking time on a daily basis to experience quiet and expanded levels of awareness in meditation is key to healing, for it is our direct opportunity to go beyond our time-bound individuality and taste our essential immortal nature. From this platform of silence, we can activate our healing intentions, through the power of prayer, ritual, or imagery. We let the cosmic forces know in no uncertain terms what we would like to happen, then we release the intention and allow nature's wisdom to work out the details.

Emotional Expression

Have the willingness, confidence, and competence to express your feelings to people willing to share in your deeply human experience of facing a life-threatening illness. It will melt the walls of alienation and isolation and provide you with access to the most profound healing force in the universe—the power of love. The healing journey is one of recognizing your universal nature. Sharing with others your hopes and disappointments, joys and sorrows, is essential to the recovery of wholeness. The support of others is a powerful healing tool, as documented by David Spiegel's work at Stanford, which showed that people participating in cancer support groups not only feel better but live longer.[7] Connect with people who can empathize with your situation and inspire you with their stories of courage and perseverance. Surround yourself with people who can cry and laugh with you, never forgetting the precious gift of life.

Family Support

When one person in a family has cancer, the whole family has cancer. Whether the dynamics of a family prior to the diagnosis were healthy or dysfunctional, serious illness shifts the entire network of relationships within a household. As is true for the individual, facing cancer provides a family with the opportunity for profound insight, wisdom, and healing. Some families naturally rally behind a loved one with a malignancy, spontaneously mixing the right blend of sadness and hope, seriousness and lightheartedness, anguish and joy, courage and surrender. For others, the fear and uncertainty surrounding cancer heightens the underlying tension and insecurities that were already straining the family bonds. Whatever existing patterns of communication predominate, cancer provides the chance to heal old wounds and establish new levels of intimacy. Yet it takes a concerted and unified effort to seize the opportunity for transformation.

Family dynamics are challenged when the family member facing cancer has traditionally been the primary caregiver. If Mom, who always nurtured everyone else, is now in need of support, other family members must rise to the occasion, *and* Mom needs to allow others to nurture her. Open and honest communication is the essential key, allowing for loved ones to make the transition into new roles.

I recommend that the family meet together on a regular basis, with each member taking turns practicing conscious communication. Allow time for each person to express their fears and hopes, recognizing that there are no right or wrong feelings. If a family member who is overwhelmed by the illness does not seem capable of carrying his or her full share of responsibilities, negotiate a role that allows him or her to make some contribution without feeling guilty for not doing more. Each of us processes loss at our own pace. If we allow people to give what they can, they will often be able to access greater inner resources as their confidence grows. Simply allowing people to express their fears and concerns will often dissipate the pressure that escalates to a fight-or-flight response. A script for a healthy family discussion may sound like the following:

MOM: I know that my breast cancer is scary for all of us. We have a difficult challenge ahead of us, but I know that if we are there for each other, we can get through this together.

DAD: We've all depended upon Mom to take care of all of us, and the thought of her really needing *us* now may be overwhelming. I'm going to make a commitment to come home a little earlier from work every day so I can help out around the house. Although I'm frightened, I'm also confident that we can weather this storm together and be a stronger family as a result of this.

14−YEAR-OLD JESSICA: It just doesn't seem fair to me! Everything was going so well in our lives and now this happens. What happens if you die? I just want to run away.

MOM: I know it doesn't seem fair, but life does not always go the way we plan it. I'm not planning on checking out anytime soon, and now I need you to be there for me. I can handle your sadness and your frustration, but please do not withdraw from me.

17−YEAR-OLD MICHAEL: Maybe I shouldn't go away to college next year so I can stay close to you. I can start at the local community college and transfer when you are feeling better.

MOM: I appreciate your offer, but I think it is too early for you to start changing your life plans. Let's proceed with the assumption that I am going to navigate my way through this challenge and you are going to attend the school that is best for you.

DAD: Does everyone feel they've had the opportunity to say what's on their mind?

JESSICA: I'm sorry that I came across as being selfish. I'm just so worried about losing Mom.

MOM: You can never really lose me, and I deeply appreciate it that you are willing to share your true feelings with me.

For the first few months after learning of the diagnosis, I strongly encourage you to have weekly family meetings to allow all family members to express themselves honestly and openly. The skills developed in such loving discussions will serve them throughout their lifetime. Having a formally scheduled powwow provides the family with a healthy mechanism for processing the strong feelings that invariably arise when serious illness intrudes. As the medical situation stabilizes, call your family meetings whenever an issue arises that is best addressed in an open forum. Empower your family members to call a meeting when they feel the strong need to express themselves. Create some ritual—saying a prayer, reading a poem—at the beginning and end of the gathering to define the experience as important and special.

If you are the person facing cancer, tell your loved ones how you would like them to treat you, acknowledging that your needs may change from day to day and during the course of your illness. The only certain way for your family to know what you want is for you to tell them. It's not fair to become upset with your loved ones for not being able to read your mind. As mentioned earlier in this chapter, some people with cancer may have difficulty expressing their needs, but this is definitely the time to change that pattern. If your family has never been that skilled at communicating, consider asking for professional help from a family counselor, minister, priest, or rabbi. Cancer gives us the opportunity to look life in the face, experience the precious gift that it is, and express our appreciation for the fleetingly brief time we have to spend together. Seize the opportunity to deepen your intimacy with your family and friends who are your fellow travelers.

As you progress in your recovery from cancer, the intensity of your feelings may diminish and your relationships with those closest to you will shift again. Family members who found themselves able to give more than they thought themselves capable of will gradually need to pull back a bit so you don't feel smothered. On the other hand, having successfully met the challenge of cancer, you will always carry the memory and wounds of the illness, and you may not want everyone else to completely forget the battle you have waged as they get on with their normal lives. As with every aspect of life, the challenge facing you and your family with cancer is to achieve the correct balance, realizing that it will always be a dynamic equilibrium.

Accurate Information and Appropriate Medical Interventions

Learning about the cancer you are facing can be very empowering. Use the world of scientific medicine for your best benefit. You are *the* critical member of the health care team and are capable of understanding everything that is known about your illness. Question, challenge, and debate with your doctor on important aspects of your care. Avoid the temptation to use denial to evade effective treatments, and be conscious of your use of magical thinking, such as "I can avoid my breast surgery if I just take these Chinese herbs for a few weeks." On the other hand, do not accept your role as a passive receptacle of modern medical pharmaceuticals.

In this information age, it is easy to become an expert in your illness. Spend a day at your local medical library, or access information from the Internet. One of the frequently cited benefits of support groups is the information available from other participants equally invested in learning as much as possible about the illness. Try to keep a balanced perspective, weighing each new approach in both your heart and mind. If a new treatment becomes available, ask to speak directly to others who have experienced it before flying across the world pursuing a legendary therapy.

If the distress of cancer is too formidable and you find yourself feeling despair, discuss the role of antidepressant medicines with your doctor. Appropriately used medications can be powerful tools in relieving the feelings of hopelessness and helplessness that interfere with your ability to elicit an optimal healing response. I view the development of effective chemotherapy drugs, potent pain relievers, and mood-enhancing medicines with the same reverence that I honor medicinal herbs, meditation, and healing touch. Choose your helping allies consciously, remembering that the true healer is not an outside agent but the powerful force within you.

Diving Deeper

For most people with cancer, there will be a stage in their healing journey when some of the intense turbulence has subsided and there is an opportunity for deeper reflection on the meaning of illness and the meaning of life. This is a time when personal transformation is possible if we are able to look honestly and openly at the choices we have made in the past and consider whether we are prepared to make different choices to create a different future. We are the sum total of the choices we have made, and serious illness allows us the opportunity to recreate ourselves in a new image, if we so desire and are willing to do the work. The "work" means looking into our hearts, seeing what is unresolved, and taking steps to release feelings and beliefs that are limiting the full expression of our higher self.

I believe there are three major components to this process that catalyze deeper understanding and personal transformation: *forgiveness, meaning*, and *vision*. Forgiveness is the reclaiming of our innocence, our natural state of being before we learned that the world was a dangerous place and that unconditional love was a rare commodity. Along our life path, we have all been hurt, disappointed, and betrayed. Most of us at some point have hurt, disappointed, and betrayed others. It is a rare person who does not carry some unhealed wound in his or her heart. And it is often the person that we have consciously rejected the most for whom we feel the deepest unspoken desire for their love and forgiveness.

Sharon had not seen her father since he left the family when she was seven years old. Her mother's rage at his abandonment was contagious, so that by the time she was a teenager any thought of him teemed with anger and resentment. When she learned that he had remarried and started a new family, Sharon vowed that she would never forgive him.

She was, therefore, fully unprepared when several years later while a freshman in college, she received a letter from him asking if she would visit. He had recently been diagnosed with pancreatic cancer and wanted to see her before he died. Although her initial reaction was to reject him the way she had been rejected, a soft but persistent inner voice compelled her to go. When, several weeks later, she encountered the frail man in his hospital bed, a flood of emotions engulfed her as he expressed his remorse and love for her. She was overwhelmed with a mixture of sadness and joy when he told her that he had been writing for years, but his letters had been returned by her mother, who felt he had no right to intrude on her life. When they parted that day, Sharon realized that her anger was her walled-off pain that had no healthy outlet for expression.

Serious illness is a reminder that we are on this earth for only a short time and that holding resentments, hurts, and grudges is a tragic waste of time and life energy. If you agree that letting go of emotional pain is desirable at this stage of your life, set aside some time when you will not be interrupted and proceed with the following exercise.

1. Meditate in silence for about ten minutes, using either breathing awareness or a mantra meditation technique.
2. Visualize a beautiful, safe, and serene environment in your mind. Choose some natural place that you associate with a time of comfort and joyfulness.

3. Envision yourself in your most divine form. It may be as an angelic being, a sagacious man or woman, or an innocent, wise child.
4. Now in this sacred space, ask yourself what resentments, old hurts, anger, or regrets you are carrying in your heart.
5. With your intention to be completely honest and open with yourself, allow your memory to carry you back through your life, recalling episodes when your heart closed down as a result of some insensitivity or betrayal by another person.
6. Recall times when you were insensitive or harsh to another person who wanted or needed attention or caring that you were unable to provide.

Spend some time writing about what you learned in this process. Recall the circumstances and feelings that came to mind and write about them freely without trying to filter the memories or emotions that rise to the surface of your awareness. When you feel complete with this "recall" part of the process, go back into meditation for five to ten minutes and again visualize your sacred space. This time ask yourself the following questions:

1. What is necessary for me to forgive others for the hurt they have caused me?
2. What is necessary for me to forgive myself for the hurt I have caused others?
3. What is necessary for me to forgive myself for the hurt I have caused myself?

Again, spend some time writing about what you have discovered in this process. Give yourself the space to digest the information and feelings that may rise to the surface. Allow yourself several days to process your emotions before acting on anything that may have been revealed. If you feel the urge to write a letter or call someone from your past that you have been resenting, wait until some of the emotional charge has subsided before acting on the impulse. Remember that you may be ready to forgive and forget, but the other person may not be. The most powerful healing takes place within your heart, regardless of how another person responds.

It is not uncommon for someone to discover they have been harboring emotional pain created by someone who is no longer alive. It may be an invalidating parent or an ex-spouse who betrayed you. If you feel ready to release toxic feelings for someone who has passed on, a ritual can be very beneficial in allowing you to complete your release. After identifying the feelings, witnessing the sensations, expressing them in writing, and releasing them with a physical process, design a ceremony that has meaning for you. Write a letter and burn it while offering your forgiveness to the person's spirit. Make a trip to their gravesite and pour out your pain, leaving something to commemorate your visit. If there are surviving family members with whom you would like to heal, such as children of an estranged sibling, write to them expressing your desire to make peace. Be creative, knowing that if you are coming from a place of love, you can only gain in the process.

Many people find it more difficult to forgive themselves for past indiscretions than to forgive others. I have found three components important to facilitating a genuine release of guilt and remorse. First, remember that everyone is doing his or her best at any moment in time. In retrospect, you may wonder in disbelief at how you could have said or done something that caused hurt to another or to yourself, but at the time of the event, you were acting with as much consciousness as was available to you. Second, perform some action to make amends—write a letter, make a donation, volunteer your services. In the process of openly giving from your heart, your heart will provide the forgiveness you seek. Finally, make the commitment not to repeat the same actions that caused the hurt. Vow to the best of your abilities to be more truthful, caring, sensitive, honest, generous, loyal, or forthright. In your promise to change, forgiveness dawns.

Finding Meaning in Illness

When encountering adversity, one of our first impulses is to ask, "Why is this happening to me?" The idea that the universe is random and capricious is unacceptable to my psyche, and yet, more often than not, I am incapable of fully answering the "why" questions. In the Vedic tradition, the expression "Unfathomable is the field of karma" recognizes that the multitude of past choices that conspired to create our current circumstance are beyond any person's ability to fully comprehend. It may seem easy to explain the lung cancer of the person who smoked for forty years, but even this simplistic idea of cause and effect raises many more questions than answers. Why did the person start in the first place? What need was the habit fulfilling? Why did the cancer arise five years after the person stopped smoking? Our ability to explain cancer in the pediatric population becomes even less conceivable as we see innocent children develop leukemia or a neuroblastoma as a result of no apparent choices they made. The book of Job in the Old Testament reminds us that bad things do happen to good people.

Even if we fail to understand why something painful has arisen, we can still find meaning in the situation. Creating meaning is a distinctly human need that must be fulfilled in order for us to continue on our path. We cannot change the past that presented us with the challenge we are facing, but we can reinterpret the experience from the perspective of life as a learning journey. As the great writer and philosopher Aldous Huxley once said, "Experience is not what happens to you. It's what you do with what happens to you."

Asking the right questions can help unveil the deeper significance of illness. These exercises, like those described earlier in this chapter, are of greatest value when you designate a time to focus on the questions, ensuring that you will not be interrupted or disturbed. Begin the process with ten minutes of meditation, allowing your mental turbulence to subside. Then visualize your inner sacred space, invoking the highest aspect of your being to facilitate your exploration of these sensitive issues. When you are ready to listen to your innermost voice, ask yourself the following questions:

1. If I knew that I had only one more year to live, what changes would I make in my life now?
2. If I were able to speak directly to my cancer, what positive message would it have for me?
3. Imagining that it is five years from now and my illness is behind me, what would I tell someone else in my situation about the meaning of my illness?
4. If I were able to speak directly to my God, what would he or she say to me about the meaning of my illness?

Begin the conversation with your inner self and listen to the messages that arise. Many people that I see at the Chopra Center discover that their cancer is providing an opportunity to make choices that bring love, intimacy, and spirituality and to no longer tolerate circumstances that are not elevating to the human spirit. The undeniable reality of life is that death is stalking every one of us, although most of us choose to live as if we have all the time in the world. If we really understood how brief and precious the human experience is, we would not waste a moment on mundane actions, resentments, or regrets. Facing cancer is an opportunity to look mortality in the face and choose the eternal present moment.

Envisioning the Future

It is common parlance in New Age circles to hear that we create our own reality. This is true to the extent that our choices define a certain set of probabilities. If I hadn't chosen to go to medical school years ago, I would probably not be writing this book today. If I had chosen to move to Texas instead of California, I would probably not have my position as medical director of the Chopra Center. On the other hand, when it comes to illness, I believe that it is an extremely rare person who consciously chooses to get sick. You may have made choices in the past that increased your probability of illness, but you did not opt for a bout with cancer.

You do have a choice about what to do next. Creating a persuasive vision of the future can have a powerful effect on your quality of life. Get clear on your intentions for the next six months, twelve months, five years. What do you want your life to look like? Consider the various aspects of your life and create a compelling future for yourself. Using the process that is by now familiar to you, spend ten minutes meditating, then visit your sacred space, envisioning yourself in the future. What will your physical, emotional, material, and professional life be like? How will your relationships feel? How will your spiritual life look?

Only you can answer these questions for yourself. Think and write about the life you would like to create and put your attention on your desires at the beginning of your daily meditations and before you go to bed at night. Write out a list of your desires and read it over several times each day. In general, it is best to keep your intentions in the quiet of your own awareness, for the delicate seeds of desires sprout most readily in silence.

If you anticipate passing on in the foreseeable future, then consider how you would like to spend your final days. Where would you like to be? Who would you like to have around you? What do you want to say in your final moments to the people you love? These are not the kinds of questions that most of us are accustomed to asking. Perhaps you are afraid to create an expectation for your future when your health seems so precarious. Perhaps you cannot think about more than one day at a time. Perhaps you are afraid to acknowledge unfulfilled desires when you are uncertain whether you will have the opportunity to realize them. All of these concerns are legitimate and, I would suggest, not that different from the concerns of people who are not facing a serious illness. However, it has been my experience that most people who are confronting the possibility of their death have a deep intuitive sense of the course of their illness. Time and again I have cared for people who knew they were going to outlive the expectations the medical establishment had for them. Other times, people were ready to let go and, even though they had no imminent reason to die, passed on quickly and peacefully.

The value of our earthly experience is not weighed by quantity but quality. I encourage you to look within your heart and listen to the quiet voice that is guiding you to wholeness. Clear away the toxic emotions that are clouding your vision of your essential divinity. Whether you live for another fifty years or soon pass on to the next phase of your journey, release your resentments and judgments so that your heart can overflow with love and forgiveness.

Commitment to Wholeness

Our bodies are the end products of our experiences and interpretations. To change our bodies, we need to change our experiences. Make a commitment to change your life in the direction of greater love and caring for yourself and those close to you.

1. I commit to taking responsibility for my feelings, choosing to view emotional challenges as opportunities for personal insight and growth.

2. I commit to releasing toxic emotions from my heart so that I can freely love and appreciate the people in my life and myself.

3. I commit to open and honest communication with the people in my life, using the challenge of cancer to deepen my connections with those I love.

CHAPTER 11

Healing through Expression

*Deepening Insight through
Drawing and Movement*

Art is the accomplice of love.
Take love away and there is no longer art.
—REMY DE GOURMONT

O body swayed to music, O brightening glance,
How can we know the dancer from the dance?
—WILLIAM BUTLER YEATS

Jennifer had learned to use her physical attractiveness since her teenage years. Although bright with a whimsical sense of humor, she privately attributed her success as a sales representative to her ability to attract potential customers with her natural beauty. When she lost her right breast to cancer, her self-esteem and confidence eroded, even though her reconstructive surgery was successful.

After several counseling sessions, her therapist suggested they try exploring art as a way of gaining insight into her deeper feelings. Because she had always enjoyed sketching as a girl, Jennifer was open to this new approach. Over the course of several sessions, she was asked to draw pictures. Her first assignment was to sketch herself before and after surgery. Her "before" picture illustrated an outgoing woman, in the center of many admiring men. In her "after" picture, she had a disfigured body and was alone.

In the next session, the therapist asked Jennifer to look at her face in the mirror, paying particular attention to her eyes. She then asked her to draw a portrait focusing on her inner beauty. This time Jennifer drew the face of a beautiful woman with beaming, luminous eyes.

Finally, she was asked to look at herself in a full-length mirror and draw exactly what she saw. Jennifer drew a picture of an attractive, radiant woman, comfortable with her natural beauty and no longer needing the approval of others to reinforce her sense of attractiveness or importance. In the art therapy process, she was able to see with increasing clarity her true grace, charm, and value. She released her long-standing need to receive approval for her appearance and became more appreciative of her natural inner beauty.

We have a fundamental need to express ourselves. As infants we gurgle and smile, shriek and thrash to attract the attention of parents and caregivers. As we become capable of more independent expression we find power and joy in the simple creative acts of speaking, singing, running, dancing, pounding on drums, scribbling, and coloring. At family gatherings, I watch children chasing each other, rushing from one room to the next. If I stop my three-year-old niece on the run and ask, "Why are you moving so quickly?" she looks at me with a quizzical expression. The question has no meaning to her, for she moves for the sheer joy of it. To the child, my question is the equivalent of asking, "Why are you breathing?" or "Why is your heart pumping?" The answer can only be: It is the nature of our lungs to breathe, our hearts to beat, and our bodies to move. It is our nature to express ourselves in the world.

The essence of mind-body medicine is the recognition that every experience of our lives occurs in both our minds and our bodies. Whether it is the joyful birthing of a baby, the winning of a championship sports match, the agonizing loss of a loved one, or the confronting of a serious illness, we carry the impressions of these experiences in both our mental and physical sheaths. Unresolved pain, fear, anxiety, depression, and resentment are stored in our minds and our bodies, dispensing toxicity that inhibits our ability to be fully present in the moment. In the previous chapter, I discussed ways to access these feelings through directed verbal explorations and questioning. These methods use the intellect as a doorway to the emotions, invoking the feelings carried in the body as core issues are revealed.

We can also use our senses to access stored impressions, thereby circumventing our impulse to analyze and intellectualize. Drumming, chanting, singing, dancing, drawing, and sculpting can all be powerful tools to explore deep feelings that need expression in order to be healed. All of these expressive arts therapies use one or more of the five senses to access emotional impressions stored in the body that may not be readily reachable through language. Let's explore two of these approaches in greater detail: art therapy and movement therapy.

Art Therapy

Long before human beings created written language to transmit their thoughts over time and distance, we expressed ourselves through pictures and images. Around the world, prehistoric people drew pictures on the walls and ceilings of inner caves, depicting actual or hoped-for events. Our Paleolithic ancestors probably spent a lot of time indoors during the Ice Age, giving them ample opportunity to practice their art. The ancient renderings of natural scenes found in the caves of Spain and France demonstrate the rich aesthetic sense of our earliest artists. Many anthropologists believe that in addition to their indisputable beauty, these drawings of wild animals were probably endowed with magical properties that gave hunters special powers over their potential food sources. By capturing the images of these animals with natural dyes and paints, early artists felt they were able to exercise some semblance of control over forces that often must have seemed indomitable.

In a similar way, Carl Jung believed that drawing pictures gives us access to the deeper, untamed emotional forces of our subconscious minds.[1] Often we do not have the words to capture the intensity or power of our feelings, but a visual representation can provide us with some clarity and a sense of influence over stormy emotions. Mandalas or circular visual designs connect us to deeper aspects of our nature and can be found in cultures around the world from the ancient Mayans to Tibetan tantrics to the domes of Byzantine churches. The mandala is a universal symbol that can be seen throughout nature. The circular symmetry of a snowflake, the radial pattern of a sea urchin, the balanced petals of a daisy, and the spiral arms of the Milky Way galaxy illustrate the universal expression of the center expanding outward, while the outside simultaneously seeks its return to the center. Our sustainer of life on earth, the sun, is a mandala,

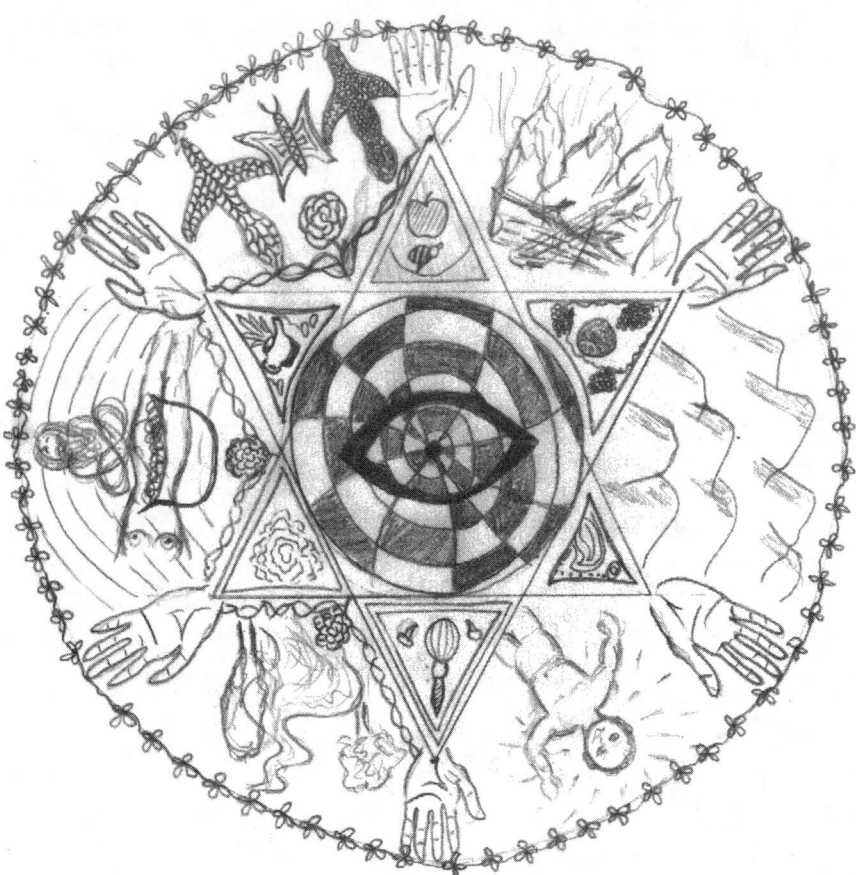

Figure 3 **Mandala**

radiating energy throughout the solar system. Some of this energy is captured by two beautiful anatomic mandalas—our eyes. Look closely at your pupils in the mirror and you will be fascinated by these living mandalas that are dancing with the light of the world.

Drawing Your Mandala

Set aside some time to draw your own mandala. When you do this exercise, plan to spend at least an hour to allow your inner images to emerge and be expressed. Gather together some drawing paper along with crayons, colored pencils, or felt-tip markers and find a space with good light that will allow you to sketch comfortably. Have a drawing compass or a string available to make circles and a straight edge to draw lines. Try the following process to help you open the portals to your inner vision.

Symbolic Journey

1. Spend ten minutes practicing a breathing awareness or mantra meditation technique.
2. Visualize your sacred space and open to the possibility that your mandala, your sacred visual symbol, is available to you in your heart of hearts.
3. Now slowly open your eyes and gather your drawing materials around you.
4. Begin by identifying the center of your page. This is the core of your being, around which all the various layers of your life are wrapped.
5. Choose any color or colors that appeal to you. Identify a space surrounding the center into which you will draw the images and impressions that express your innermost hopes and desires. It often helps to draw a light circle around the center to define this realm. Draw with an attitude of curiosity and openness without resisting or anticipating the forms that arise.
6. Moving out from the circle, sketch the images and shapes that express your emotions, feelings, and beliefs about your current life circumstance.
7. Continuing to expand your mandala, depict the images that express your current physical state, allowing your drawing to visually record the messages your body is sending.
8. In the circumference of your mandala, represent your environment in symbols and forms that emerge from your source of creativity.
9. Continue adding whatever detail you are moved to render until you feel complete with the drawing.
10. Now review the images that you have produced and see what insights may dawn. Write a few paragraphs that verbally express the feelings and sensations your mandala has evoked.

The mandala is a symbol of unity and integration. It allows a conversation to take place between our innermost impulses and our conscious perceptions and interpretations. The paradox of life is how we can simultaneously exist in the eternal, unbounded, and unchanging depths of being, while in our daily lives we see ourselves moving through constant states of transition. Mandalas enable us to participate in an active visual meditation that integrates the silent and dynamic aspects of our life. In the process of rendering these diagrams, we are reminded that we are more than material forms with awareness; rather, we are awareness manifesting as extraordinary individual expressions. Mandalas remind us that our essential nature is beyond time and space, beyond health and sickness, beyond life and death.

I strongly encourage you to try this exercise. Talking about or thinking about drawing a mandala will not offer the same experience. If you have not explored this process before, I assure you that the time you take to draw your sacred symbols will be well spent. Witnessing images emerge from deeper levels of awareness is awe-inspiring. I suggest you commit to drawing a mandala once a month as a dynamic pictorial of your healing process. Your body, mind, and soul will thank you.

Illustrating a Story

The drawing of mandalas is a powerful technology to access the deeper meaning of the challenge you are facing. It is an abstract and free-form process. For some people, a more representational approach is easier. Drawing pictures of your current and desired life situation can be revealing and clarifying. If it has been a long time since you have attempted to draw, you will be pleasantly rewarded for your willingness to explore. If you are a commercial artist or an architect by profession, it may help at the beginning to use your nondominant hand. This may enable you to bypass your discerning and critical mind to access deeper images. Try the following exercise designed to illustrate your inner mind's perception of your situation.

Scenario 1

1. Gather together some colored pencils and drawing paper. Watercolors are often very helpful in releasing creative energies.
2. Spend about ten minutes in silent meditation.
3. Envision your sacred space and visualize your highest self. Call forth in your imagination the people who are most important in your life at this time—your family members, intimate friends, and health care providers.

4. Now, slowly open your eyes and begin drawing the scene that was revealed to you. Be certain to place yourself in the picture along with other members of your inner circle.
5. Continue drawing or painting until you feel complete with the scene.
6. Now notice what messages emerged from your inner mind. What are your relationships to the people in your life? What more do you need from them that you may not be currently receiving?
7. Spend some time describing and journaling your life scene and your feelings about what you have illustrated.

Scenario 2

1. Put your first picture aside and spend another ten minutes in silent meditation.
2. Again, envision entering your sacred space and invoking your highest self. Invite the important people in your life to join you in your sacred space.
3. This time imagine having a conversation with each of these important people in which you express your needs to them. Imagine that they respond in the manner that provides you with the nourishment, love, and support that you need and deserve.
4. When you are ready, open your eyes and draw in as much detail as possible the scene that you have envisioned.
5. Again, take time to write about your inner vision as depicted on paper. What is necessary for you to create the scene you desire? What is limiting your willingness to ask for the love and support you need?
6. Make a commitment to yourself to take steps to create the life scene that provides you with the greatest amount of peace, love, and comfort and wholeness.

These visual processes can be thought of as snapshots of your inner landscape. I encourage you to set aside time on a weekly basis to document your healing journey. Facing a life-threatening illness is a mythical voyage that every human being must face. Expressing yourself through art allows you to connect with the deeper forces that transcend your individuality. Birthing these images into the world can bring insight, understanding, and empowerment.

Healing Movement

Of what is the body made? It is made of emptiness and rhythm.
At the ultimate heart of the body, at the heart of the world,
there is no solidity.
Once again there is only the dance.
GEORGE LEONARD

Our psyche and our physicality are inextricably interwoven. According to Ayurveda, our breath is the link between the mind and the body. Our first inhalation marks the formal starting point for our earthly individuality, which continues until our last exhalation releases us from our localization in time and space. All our breaths in between reflect the alchemy of consciousness transmuting into matter. The movement of breath mirrors the collective inspiration, holding, and release of every cell and tissue in our body. When we are carrying fear, anxiety, hostility, or frustration, the language of our body communicates these emotions with every breath. Listening to your body's messages and learning to release your unprocessed pain is key to healing both mind and body.

Tension-Releasing Exercise

"No matter how many times I take a deep breath, I still feel that I am not getting enough oxygen," the forty-two-year-old man with a recently diagnosed malignant melanoma complained to me. "My chest X rays, lung scans, and pulmonary function tests are all totally normal, but I feel that there is a constant weight on my chest. I know that it is related to my anxiety over this skin cancer, but I don't know what else to do about it. I don't want to take tranquilizers."

Under times of intense stress, most people project the tension they are experiencing into their bodies. For this man, the heaviness he was experiencing in his mind was causing a sense of restriction in his breathing. Reassured by his normal studies that he did not have structural problems in his heart or lungs, I instructed him in a tension-releasing exercise. As he consciously used his breath to dissipate areas of pressure in his body, he found his respiration becoming regular and effortless. I encouraged him to vocalize the sensations he was experiencing with moans and groans. After several breaths, he began sobbing as his restrained fears and grief were given permission to flow. After a thirty-minute session, he reported that "a weight had been lifted off." With further relaxation training and insight counseling, his breathing symptoms completely resolved.

A simple but powerful way to release stored emotional and physical obstructions is through the following healing exercise derived from the yoga tradition. Find a time and space where you will not be interrupted for at least thirty minutes.

1. Lie on a padded floor, cushioning your body with a thin mat or soft blanket.
2. Position yourself so that you are very comfortable. Place a small pillow or rolled towel under your neck, place pillows under your knees, and extend your arms to either side with your palms relaxed and open.
3. Now, place your attention on your breathing and with each exhalation have the intention to release any tension you are holding in your body.
4. After several minutes, shift into body awareness in which you allow your attention to go into your whole body, noticing specific areas of tension or discomfort.
5. With your attention on the area that is causing distress, begin to moan with each exhalation, imagining that the part of your body that is uncomfortable is releasing the sound along with the pain.
6. Allow your sounds to resonate throughout your body—through your belly, chest, throat, and head. Have your intention on releasing whatever sensations arise.
7. Do not resist any emotions that arise to the surface. Allow any sobbing, crying, wailing, or shrieking to be expressed, with the awareness that your mind and your body are releasing uncomfortable feelings that have been stored.
8. When the release feels complete, spend a few more minutes with your attention on your breath before opening your eyes.
9. Journal your experience and any insights that may have surfaced with this process.

Therapeutic Dance

As any pregnant mom will tell you, even in the womb we are dancing. On our first day of life we are already participating in a choreography with mother, moving in response to her words and gestures in subtle syn-chrony.[2] Our physical language expresses our emotional tone, showing restriction and tension when we are strained, and freedom, grace and flu-idity when we are comfortable. We cannot directly peer into each other's mental condition but we all announce our emotional state to the world by how we carry our bodies. Our posture, stance, and movement express the memories carried in our muscles, the earliest patterns of which were laid long ago. We carry genetic, familial, and cultural blueprints for how to position and move ourselves. We then overlay our experiences onto our physical framework. Just as changing our mood can change our body lan-guage, changing the way we use our body can have profound effects on our emotional state.

Everyone can dance. You may have been awkward or clumsy as a child, but if you are alive, you have the ability to move your body with freedom and rhythm. I encourage you to try this process, particularly if you are feeling emotionally or physically restricted. Even if you are con-fined to a chair or bed, this exercise will improve your well being.

1. Choose some music that has emotional power for you. It could be a beautiful classical piece, a New Age musical journey, or some rous-ing rock and roll. Ideally, it should be at least five minutes long and express different moods. See the reference section for a few of my suggestions.
2. If possible, have someone with whom you feel close serve as your wit-ness. A partner, family member, friend, or therapist is present to ob-serve your process and listen as you describe your experience. If you belong to a cancer support group, pairing off with another member can be a powerful way of gaining insight, sharing, bonding, and ex-pressing support.
3. Dim the lights, making certain your space is clear of obstacles.
4. Begin the process in silence, standing with your eyes closed. Allow your awareness to go into your body, feeling whatever sensations are there.
5. If there is discomfort or pain, allow your attention to acknowledge it without resistance. If there are no obvious sensations, feel the level of tension in your chest, stomach, or neck and simply allow your atten-tion to embrace whatever feelings are present. If there is no area that is capturing your awareness, see if you can feel your body pulsating with your heartbeat.
6. Now, begin your music and have the intention to allow movement to arise from the area of your body that is asking to be expressed.

7. Envision your breath flowing into the area, and as you exhale, allow any sound to emerge, using that sound as a starting point for movement.

8. Expand whatever movement is emerging. Sway, rock, swing, or twist while you maintain your awareness inside. Allow the area of pain or trauma to assert itself. If grief arises, allow it to be expressed. If anger is awakened, allow your body to deliver and liberate it. If joy and ecstasy burst forth, exalt in their declaration of independence. It's okay to have these emotions. Use movement and sound to awaken and release your unexpressed feelings.

9. When your body feels expended, find a position, sitting or lying, and become completely still. Keep your awareness inside with your eyes closed for several minutes while you observe the sensations in your body and the images in your mind.

10. Now, journal your experiences and insights and share them with your partner. Ask for observations and feedback.

A Word on Journaling

I have been encouraging you to journal in many of the exercises of this book, because I have found it to be an invaluable way to assist with personal transformation. Studies have shown that writing during difficult times improves mental and physical well being.[3] During challenging times in life, our minds and bodies strive to integrate change into our existing network of physical sensations, emotions, ideas, and desires. Most of the time we identify who we are with our bodies, feelings, and beliefs. If we are suddenly confronted with a serious illness like cancer, each of these layers is challenged, and we are forced to face new perceptions, sensations, and ideas about who we are. At first we may mobilize our defenses to avoid change, but our health is dependent upon our ability to metabolize and integrate new experiences, no matter how uncomfortable they may feel at the time. Journaling is an important way to assist this process.

The very act of writing reminds me that I am not the experiences I am having, but, rather, the silent witness to the one who is having the experiences. At one time or another, the same "I" was upset about going on a yellow school bus to my first day of kindergarten, excited about graduating from high school, grieving the loss of my sister, celebrating the birth of my children . . . and on and on. Writing about my experiences highlights the continuity of the *experiencer*, so that any particular challenging event can be viewed within the context of a bigger life.

Journaling provides form and substance to emotions and ideas. When fears and anxieties are swirling around inside, they can create a tornado of sensations that may feel overwhelming. Writing about feelings gives them expression and establishes their boundaries. You will often find that insight dawns as you attempt to define your experience within the parameters of language. Being fully present with your emotions and sensations and then writing about them is a potent combination. Then your feelings can serve their purpose of motivating changes in your life, which can ultimately offer you greater wisdom and freedom.

Moving into Wholeness

What is the value of exploring the expressive arts therapies if you are facing a life-threatening illness such as cancer? I believe there are many. The most immediate value is in bringing you into present moment awareness. When you listen to your body and allow it to speak, your mind can disengage from your usual fear-based ruminations. Opening your creative channels and allowing deeper emotions and feelings to surface bring their own rewards. With art and healing movement, we tap into images and sensations that transcend our present complex of worries and anxieties, reminding us of our connection to a source that is profoundly wise and expansive.

As we identify and release tension and restrictions from our body, we free up life energy that becomes available to us for healing and creativity. When our bodies move with greater freedom, openness, and ease, our thinking process also gains flexibility and spontaneity. We acquire a broader perspective and gain access to new creative options. A mind unfettered with discouraging thoughts is much better able to transmit healing messages to the cells and tissues of the body.

In traditional cultures around the world, the shaman or medicine man uses music, drumming, and dance to create a healing ritual. Upon a background of rhythmic beating, the spirit doctor uses primal chants and choreography to reenact ancient myths. The entire tribe participates in the ceremonial rites as patient and community unite in a healing trance. The medicine man uses all five senses to invoke images of a sacred place to which doctor and patient are transported. There, the healing wisdom of ancient spirits is imparted. Upon return to normal time and space, the mind and body of the afflicted soul have undergone a powerful transformation.

If we are uncomfortable with the thought of a healing journey to the spirit world, we can use modern terminology. When people with illness use the expressive arts therapies, they gain access to aspects of their unconscious mind where archetypal energies are available. Through the identification and release of deep-rooted emotional pain, healthier physiological and biochemical information is transmitted to their healing system. Regardless of which worldview predominates in an individual's or society's consciousness, experiencing the power of these nonverbal approaches is transformational.

Life is for learning, and for many people, learning through the body is a new and exhilarating experience. Most of us have been trained to gain knowledge through intellectual avenues, using language as the primary means to record and recall information. The expressive therapies acknowledge another primordial form of learning, which recognizes that intelligence pervades the entire body and is not just localized to the brain. The enlivening of vitality that results from giving the body the opportunity to directly express itself inspires profound healing.

Commitment to Wholeness

Our bodies are the end products of our experiences and interpretations. To change our bodies, we need to change our experiences. Make a commitment to change your life in the direction of greater love and caring for yourself and those close to you.

1. I will regularly bring my awareness to the sensations in my body, consciously attending to any messages of distress they are communicating.

2. I will provide myself opportunities to express my feelings and emotions through art, music, and dance.

3. I will begin a journal and use it to connect with, express, and release my feelings without hurting the people closest to me.

CHAPTER 12

The Best Medicine

Laughter as Therapy

Humor is a prelude to faith and Laughter is the beginning of prayer.
—Reinhold Niebuhr

Strange, when you come to think of it, that of all the countless folk who have lived before our time on this planet not one is known in history or in legend as having died of laughter.—Sir Max Beerbohm

Uncontrollable laughter arose among the blessed gods.—Homer

Laughter is the experience of the paradox of life. Our minds and our senses experience the world through the coexistence of opposites. Hot is not possible without cold, large is not conceivable without small, up has no meaning in the absence of down. We cannot know courage without fear, light without darkness, gain without loss. We can and do at times take these contradictions very seriously, for the polarities of life are the basis of tension and conflict. On the other hand, we can occasionally look at a predicament, ripe with contradictions, and burst out laughing at its absurdity. Our experience of a situation is much more dependent upon our interpretation—on our attitude—than it is on the circumstance itself. The issues of failed romance, financial struggle, and family skeletons are the substance of both soap operas and situation comedies. In one, we become engrossed in the drama, riding each wave of betrayal and reconciliation with our heart and gut. In the other, we are repeatedly pushed back from excessive intensity by an unanticipated facial expression or a witty verbal retort. A simple shift in perspective is the difference between feelings of anxiety and grief or amusement and hilarity.

When facing a serious illness, the thought of laughing at the situation may seem in itself laughable. Life does not seem even a little funny if you are feeling uncomfortable from cancer or its treatment. Yet focusing on the pain without the intention to create a shift in perspective may only intensify physical and emotional anguish. Whatever the challenge facing us, we can creatively expand our perspective and develop a different relationship to it.

> The elderly couple was receiving a tour of heaven after having been killed instantly in an automobile accident. The angel informed them that because they had lived a good life, they were being rewarded with a beautiful celestial home, a new fuel-free car, and unlimited charge accounts.
>
> Despite these boons, Mr. Newman looked distressed. "What's the problem?" his wife asked him. "Aren't you happy that we're here?"
>
> "I am," he replied, "but I can't stop thinking that if you hadn't forced me to exercise, avoid rich foods, and stop smoking my cigars, I could have been here years ago."

We have all found ourselves facing difficult circumstances with no easy solution when a good friend calls. Within a minute, our buddy has us laughing at ourselves, reminding us there is more than one way to view the situation. The very experience of laughter creates a shift in awareness and in our physical condition.

We create a reality for every scenario in our life. Our sensations and perceptions activate a network of neurological circuits that establish the limits of the experience. We become convinced that our current situation and sensations are the only possible interpretation, actually believing that our view of the world is the only correct one. Then without warning, laughter provides a brief boost to a different and greater reality. It allows us to glimpse the bigger picture, reminding us that reality is an interpretation. It is not frozen in time and space, but perpetually mutable, subject to the context of our personal and cultural memories. Laughter allows us to temporarily step outside our space and time-bound state and touch the field of awareness that is boundless and eternal.

What happens when we laugh at a scene in a film comedy? We witness a situation that usually makes us slightly uncomfortable because we can identify with the vulnerabilities of the characters. Then someone says or does something that uncovers the hidden conversation that has been taking place, we suddenly shift in our point of view, and we feel internally tickled. A connection is made between the predictable way of looking at the situation and an offbeat way. As human beings, the experience of this connection feels good and makes us laugh.

> A financially successful president of a major corporation had no grandchildren from his three married sons, despite several years of not-too-subtle coaxing. At the start of a family dinner with his sons and their spouses in attendance, the father closed his eyes and began saying grace.
>
> "Dear heavenly Father, I have received many blessings, but still, I have no grandchildren. I so desired to see my name carried into the next generation that several years ago I started a trust fund for my first grandchild, which is now worth several million dollars. I hope, with your grace, that before I die, I will have the joy of giving this gift." When the father opened his eyes, his wife was the only person remaining at the dinner table.

Humor affords us the opportunity to look at life's challenges while maintaining some detachment. When characters in a sitcom lose their jobs or find themselves in complicated love triangles, we laugh at their struggles to resolve their conflicts, because they are not *our* conflicts. This doesn't mean that we are taking pleasure in the fact that these characters are having problems. We do this in other venues, such as adventure or drama stories in which we are glad when the villain gets his due. But in comedies, we take pleasure because the character's problems are *not* our problems. In fact, if we go to a comedy film which is about a topic that is "too close to home," we may not find it funny, even though others who can identify with the issues find it hysterical.

Ultimate freedom dawns when we are able to laugh at ourselves. The ego is consumed with issues of control and approval and, as such, takes itself very seriously. The ego lives in fear of loss. The spirit is eternally free of such fears, for it knows itself as infinite and timeless. Spirit is the ground of existence, eternally taking on disguises of individuality. It rejoices in the limitless variety of expressions as it rejoices in the underlying unity. When we have spirit established as our internal reference point, we can laugh at our attachment to the confined image of ourselves.

When I realize that the real me is not those things that I identify with in my day-to-day existence—my possessions, my positions, my name, even my body—but the field of awareness that underlies all these things, laughter bubbles up inside of me. If I can have the same detachment to my own predicament as I have when watching Charlie Chaplin or Robin Williams cope with their fanciful lives, I can choose my perspective. One day I may favor seeing my challenge as a drama, another day it may be as an adventure, and on other days it may be a comedy. Whatever my choice, I will not have surrendered my freedom in the process.

Our Natural State

According to some religious traditions, human beings are born into a state of sin. However, when I watch my three-month-old baby girl spontaneously smile and laugh out loud, I have trouble believing that God did not intend for us to enjoy the goodness of life. My little Sara seems to smile for no apparent reason at all. When I smile back at her, she escalates to the next level, promptly giggling and flailing her limbs as if the entire universe was cracking up with her. I have seen reports that babies smile thirty-five times more often than adults and laugh aloud several times an hour. What are they smiling and laughing at? We'll never know for sure, as most of us have forgotten, but I suspect they're laughing because it simply feels good to be alive. In addition, it feels good to laugh, thereby completing a perfect resonating loop.

No matter how seriously I might be concerned about something, when I see my daughter chuckling away, I am compelled to join in her laughter. The critically important issue I was occupied with did not change, but my perspective shifted. And serendipitously, from my new viewpoint, previously unrecognized solutions often come to light. Laughter can be healing and enlightening. One of the many gifts our children offer us is the reminder not to take ourselves so seriously.

The Science of Humor

Two men had been in business together for over thirty years when one came down with an illness that defied diagnosis and treatment. As he was lying on his deathbed, his conscience got the better of him and he called in his longtime associate. "I have to admit something to you before I die," the sick man lamented, "I don't want to take this to my grave. The truth is I've been embezzling money from our company for the past twenty years and have probably stolen over a million dollars from you. I beg that you'll forgive me before I die."

"Don't be too hard on yourself," the healthy partner quickly responded. "I too have been self-serving. To tell you the truth, it's me who's been poisoning you for the past six months."

From a scientific perspective, laughter is an elegant and complex mind-body phenomenon. Your daughter's giggles as you tickle her are expressing a response that has many psychological and neurological components. The sensation of tickling under her arms is carried by nerve fibers to different levels of the brain, triggering a host of reactions. Messages to her arms and legs cause her to squirm. Neurological inputs to her breathing muscles and voice box stimulate the sounds and exhalations of laughter. If your tickling is unrelenting, impulses may travel to her lacrimal glands, resulting in tears of joy. All the while, her interpretation of the experience is key. If she did not perceive the tickling as safe, a whole different set of responses would be evoked. If she is mad at you because you made her leave her friend's party before she wanted to, she may determinedly suppress her giggling despite your valiant efforts to evoke it.

Although my spaniel seems to smile when I scratch her belly, only human beings laugh. (Hyenas are not really laughing but producing an unusual bark to define their personal space.) Babies are able to smile within their first month of life but aren't able to laugh until the third or fourth. Studies in the first half of the twentieth century documented the developmental history of smiling and laughing in children. At eighteen months of age, we smile about every six minutes, but by age four we are grinning almost once per minute. Similarly the ratio of laughs to smiles increases from one in ten at a year and a half to one laugh for every three smiles when we are four years old.[1] Other studies correlate intelligence with the frequency of laughter.[2]

Sometimes we laugh because we hear something clever, and sometimes we laugh because we see something incongruous, as when an authority figure gets locked in a closet, or a policeman slips on a banana peel. My best laughs come when I can't really figure out what's so funny. I usually notice this when at a later time I try to explain the reason for my mirth to someone else and it invariably fails to reproduce the effect. Laughter can be contagious, as most of us have experienced at one time or another. We begin laughing just because someone else is and find ourselves caught in a self-perpetuating circuit, in which we continue laughing just thinking about how hard we've been laughing.

Despite the ubiquitous experience of laughter, scientific research into its medicinal value is relatively sparse. Almost five hundred years ago, the French physician and humorist François Rabelais saw that laughter was therapeutic: "It is better to write about laughter than tears, For laughter is the property of man."[3]

Norman Cousins, author and editor of *Saturday Review*, brought laughter to the forefront with his book *Anatomy of an Illness*, published in 1979. In it he recounts how he was able to recover from a rare and usually progressive arthritic condition by mobilizing his healing energies through laughter and vitamin C. He would watch old *Candid Camera* and Marx Brothers films, finding that a "dose" of a belly laugh would provide two hours of pain relief.[4, 5] Other than disturbing other patients with his chuckling, the laughter produced only positive side effects. Within days he was sleeping better, and his laboratory studies confirmed that the inflammation in his body was subsiding. Over a period of months his mobility improved, and after several years, he made an almost complete recovery.

Over the past few years, research has confirmed that laughing produces beneficial physiological changes. Laughter reduces the output of stress hormones and increases the vitality of natural killer cells.[6] Watching an hour-long humorous video can increase your blood level of the natural immune-enhancing chemical gamma-interferon for nearly a day.[7] In Japan people with rheumatoid arthritis who watched "rakugo," or traditional comic storytelling, had a significant reduction in their pain and stress hormones levels along with rises in two immune-enhancing chemicals.[8] Humor can reduce anxiety, soften anger, lighten depression, and raise our tolerance for pain.[9-11] In all seriousness, laughter is good for our body, mind, and soul.

Invoking Laughter

A noticeably agitated man entered the psychiatrist's office.

"I think I'm going crazy," he blurted out. "I'm having recurrent dreams and obsessive thoughts about Native American culture."

"Tell me about them," the psychiatrist encouraged.

"Well, I know it sounds bizarre," the patient responded hesitantly, "but sometimes I imagine I'm a teepee and others times I fantasize that I'm a wigwam."

"Don't worry," the psychiatrist reassured the man, "you're not going crazy. You're just too tense."

Talking about the value of laughter is about as fulfilling as talking about eating a delicious, nutritious feast or the enjoyment of making love. Ultimately, the benefit is not in the description but in the experience. As human beings, we are continuously facing the challenges life offers us, and they often feel overwhelming. What can we as human beings do to bring more levity into our lives so we can face these challenges with grace and wisdom?

Laughter is a communal, as well as a personal, experience. We usually laugh more when others are laughing with us. This is why we hear canned laugh tracks on every television sitcom. I encourage you to go to movies, plays, and comedy shows where you can be swept up in collective mirth. Look for humor in your life and give yourself permission to laugh out loud when something strikes your funny bone. Expose yourself to situations that will tickle your sense of humor. Here are a few suggestions:

~   Make funny faces at your family and friends.
~   Visit a park and observe children and dogs playing.
~   Watch old comedy films.
~   Have a staring contest with your friend.
~   Watch television comedy reruns from your childhood.
~   Start a pillow fight.
~   Instigate a food fight (marshmallows are fun without being messy).
~   Read joke books.
~   Jump in puddles.
~   Blow bubbles.
~   Twirl a hula hoop.
~   Call an old high school friend.
~   Dodge the ocean waves.
~   Go to an amusement park.

Be creative. Think about times in your life when you were carefree and lighthearted and recreate those experiences. Remember that you don't need to be in a good mood all the time. You just need to have a good belly laugh once a day.

Laughing Meditation

The great Tantric sage Osho believed in making all of life a meditation. Breathing, talking, eating, walking—with awareness any experience could be a means to higher consciousness. One of his many meditations used laughing to cleanse the heart and access the soul.[12] I have personally used this technique and can attest to its transformational effect. This exercise is particularly powerful when performed in groups, but is also very effective if you are by yourself. To begin the process, find a comfortable space and just start laughing out loud. At first it will feel contrived, but within a few minutes, your body will take over and laughter will bubble up for no reason other than the sheer joy of it. Use funny gibberish words to get yourself going, or use the expression suggested by Osho, "Yaa-Hoo!" After twenty to thirty minutes of hysterical laughing, lie absolutely quietly and release any emotions that arise. You may find that a wave of sadness wells up, emancipated by the laughter. Allow your feelings to flow, relinquishing the need to analyze or judge them.

Laughing

But seas do laugh, show white, when rocks are near.
JOHN WEBSTER

Laughing in the face of adversity is a supreme challenge. It requires a heroic effort, but I believe we all have the potential to be heroes and heroines in the drama of life. Facing a life-threatening illness demands that we look seriously at our choices, and then in the most lighthearted manner, relinquish our attachment to our self-image, allowing our true self to be expressed.

In my favorite novel, *Jitterbug Perfume*, author Tom Robbins describes our final scene as individuals. We come before an ethereal being who oversees a brass scale, on which one balance sits a hawk feather. The being reaches into our chest and removes our heart, which is placed on the other balance. The dialogue continues:

> "We weigh their hearts. Should a person possess a heart that is as light as a feather, then that person is granted immortality."
> "Indeed? Are there many?"
> "Few, precious few, I am sorry to say. One would think that people would catch on. Those who pass the test are usually rather odd. . . . The ordinary rarely beat the scales."[13]

Perhaps the greatest gift we can offer those we love is a regular reminder not to take themselves too seriously. The goal of life may be to lighten up, despite the gravity that pervades this plane of existence. Perhaps this is why the wise sages refer to the ultimate state of liberation as enlightenment.

Commitment to Wholeness

Our bodies are the end products of our experiences and interpretations. To change our bodies, we need to change our experiences. Make a commitment to change your life in the direction of greater love and caring for yourself and those close to you.

1. I will look for the humor in life and allow myself to laugh freely and heartily at every opportunity.

2. I will make responsible choices to bring healing influences into my life, but I will try not to take myself too seriously.

3. I will give myself permission to commit acts of silliness, irresponsibility, and lightheartedness on a daily basis. I will relinquish the belief that being mature means being sullenly serious.

CHAPTER 13

Weighing the Options

Assessing and Utilizing Alternative Medicine

I will prescribe regimen for the good of my patients according to my ability and my judgment and never do harm to anyone.—THE HIPPOCRATIC OATH

The worst medical experience I can remember was a middle-aged lady who came to the emergency room with her first epileptic seizure. By the time she arrived, she had fully regained consciousness and wanted to go home, but the neurology resident insisted that she undergo a CT scan of the brain before she left. She argued with him, insisting that she did not believe in medical doctors and wanted to talk with her chiropractor before any tests were done. The young doctor, who acknowledged the value of alternative doctors, voiced his strong opinion that a chiropractor knew nothing about epilepsy and warned that she was risking her well being by forgoing the brain scan. After the doctor's strong admonition to the patient and her family, she reluctantly agreed to proceed with the scan.

A few minutes later, the radiologist called the neurology resident, saying that the plain pictures raised the possibility of a small brain tumor and recommended that intravenous contrast dye be given to better clarify the lesion. The resident agreed and began walking to the radiology suite to review the films. Just as he was entering the department, he heard, "Code blue team to the CT room! Code blue team to the CT room!" blasting from the hospital

195

intercom system. As he rushed to the scanner, he saw his patient in full cardiac arrest, undergoing CPR. Despite an hour of intensive resuscitative efforts, she was pronounced dead, the result of a severe allergic reaction to the dye.

This experience is etched into my memory because I was the neurology resident who insisted on the scan. I remember this scene because I believe it was the day that my smug medical doctor ego received its fatal wound. Like most products of medical school, I was raised on the dogma that M.D.s are the only *real* doctors and all others are imposters. We talk about Western medicine as "traditional," even though it is one of the newest systems on the health care scene. We disparage other healing systems as alternative, unconventional, or unproven, despite information that between one-third and one-half of all Americans routinely seek care from alternative providers,[1, 2] and more than half of people with cancer undergo "unorthodox" treatments.[3] We take pride in our scientific war on cancer, highlighting recent slight declines in the incidence and death rates for certain cancers.[4] And yet, it is important to recognize that the bulk of our incremental success is due primarily to prevention and early detection. It remains unclear whether our advanced cancer treatments are having a substantial health impact, despite twenty-five years and $25 billion of research.[5]

Many people facing cancer are drawn to metabolic therapies, strict diets, megavitamins, and shark cartilage because they believe these treatments are helpful and they fulfill a need that is not met by conventional cancer treatments. Alternative interventions are usually without serious side effects and offer hope when standard treatments have failed. As a cancer patient, you have almost certainly been encouraged by a friend or family member to seek some type of alternative care. On one hand, you don't want to ignore an opportunity that may add quality or quantity to your life. On the other, you wouldn't consciously choose to waste time and money on a treatment that is unlikely to provide any benefit. This important issue of unproven therapies often creates additional anguish in people facing cancer, in part because of the extreme polarization that surrounds alternative approaches. In this chapter, I'll share my honest, and hopefully balanced, perspective on how I assess the vast array of alternative interventions. Ultimately, the decision to explore an alternative treatment is a personal one, but I believe there are some basic principles that can make your choice easier.

What Is Alternative?

A twenty-eight-year-old woman with Hodgkin's lymphoma told me, "I want to do everything possible to beat this disease. My herbalist told me I should be taking Essiac, my chiropractor wants me to take ozone therapy, and my nutritionist is encouraging me to go macrobiotic. When I ask one of my advisors about advice the other one is providing, they tell me I need to decide for myself if I think their recommendations are helpful. I wouldn't dare mention these other approaches to my oncologist, who thinks they are all a waste of time and money."

When I asked her how she was feeling with all these holistic interventions, she replied, "Confused. I really don't know if anything is helping but I am afraid to stop anything in case it is."

Unfortunately, the above story is a common one. There are so many different approaches available today that it is nearly impossible for most people to sort out what is valuable and what is rumor. Even as medical director of the Chopra Center, where I am constantly being introduced to new treatments, I have difficulty keeping up with the science, let alone the mystical cures that are so elusive to pin down. In this section, I hope to provide you with an approach that will allow you to rationally assess alternative interventions. I believe it is essential that you maintain responsibility for the choices you make and not surrender your authority to an "expert," just because they are promising you the dramatic result you've been hoping for.

In my mind, a treatment is not "alternative" just because it has its roots in another culture or medical tradition. Ginger has been scientifically shown to reduce the symptoms of motion sickness; therefore, this traditional herbal remedy is no more alternative than the drug meclizine.[6] Since massage has been demonstrated to improve outcomes in premature babies, there is no logical reason that it should be considered alternative.[7] How or why a therapeutic intervention works often takes much longer to understand than the recognition that a treatment is beneficial. Doctors knew that aspirin was effective in reducing fever, pain, and inflammation long before we discovered prostaglandins. It's reassuring to have a rational explanation for a treatment's efficacy, but the absence of one does not preclude its potential benefit. As a medical doctor I feel much more comfortable prescribing a chili pepper cream for diabetic nerve pain, knowing that the spicy fruit contains a chemical, capsaicin, that depletes tiny nerve endings of a pain-inducing peptide. However, I am not justified in rejecting a treatment just because I don't understand the mechanism of its action.

As a discerning person, I do need to hear some potentially rational argument as to why something might be helpful. For some alternative approaches, there are important basic assumptions, which if accepted lead to logical explanations for their efficacy. In Traditional Chinese Medicine, energy (chi) is believed to circulate through channels known as meridians. Illness can result from blocked channels; therefore, placing acupuncture needles into specific sites can release the blockage and restore health. Western science may develop other explanations for the efficacy of acupuncture in terms of gate theories or endorphin release. In either case, there is an inherent consistency, even as we are trying to bridge the two different paradigms.

With other alternative therapies, explanations can sometimes seem logical but are based upon a theory that uses bad science. For example, proponents of the Gerson program and its derivatives promote coffee enemas as an important component of their detoxification process. They propose that coffee stimulates enzymes in the liver that neutralize free radicals and that these neutralized toxins are converted into bile salts that can then be flushed out of the gallbladder. The difficulty with this explanation is that coffee has never been shown to have this effect.[8] It's a fascinating theory, but one without scientific basis. This doesn't negate the value of other components of the program such as eliminating tobacco and cigarettes and the favoring of a vegetarian diet, but it makes it difficult for a scientist to trust the integrity of the program.

The major problem with most alternative cancer treatments is the almost complete lack of controlled clinical trials to support their value. What is the difference between claims for an extract of the Pacific yew tree (taxol) and claims for the derivative of apricot pits (laetrile)? Randomized trials documented benefits for taxol, which could not be shown for laetrile.[9, 10] Although some alternative cancer treatment proponents raise the flag of a cancer industry conspiracy to suppress effective treatments, I don't buy into that. Like most physicians I know, I recognize the limitations of modern cancer treatments. And although I would like to believe that some very simple natural approach could completely eliminate cancer without any side effects, I have yet to see such a program.

As a resident in internal medicine at the University of California at San Diego Medical Center, I saw many patients transferred on an emergency basis to our medical unit who had traveled long distances to receive treatment at laetrile clinics in Tijuana, Mexico, or alternative cancer centers in San Diego County. I shared firsthand the anguish of these people who had been unsuccessfully treated by standard and alternative medicine. Although I completely understand the intense need to do *something* when modern medicine offers limited efficacy, I believe it is essential that people with cancer and their devoted families have a framework for evaluating the claims of unproven therapies.

Asking the Questions

Since it is unlikely that any alternative treatment meets the stringent guidelines for scientific efficacy (if it did, it would no longer be alternative), how can we assess the value of these therapies? There are many questions I find helpful when trying to learn about a new cancer treatment:

~   What are the claims being made for the treatment?
~   What is the rationale for the treatment?
~   How well documented are the cases that are used to support the treatment efficacy?
~   How long have the patients been followed since they underwent the alternative therapy?
~   How much does the treatment cost?
~   What are the side effects of the treatment?

It is unlikely that these questions will be fully answerable for most alternative cancer treatments, but you can usually get a good sense about the integrity of the program and the people promoting it. Let's go into each question in more detail.

What are the claims being made for the treatment?

The adage that if something sounds too good to be true, it probably is, applies well to cancer treatments. Is the program promising a cure for your illness, or are they suggesting improvement in your quality of life? Does the program claim successful experience with thousands of patients, or does it acknowledge that some people improve and some do not? Regardless of what expectations are being created, ask to communicate directly with several former clients, preferably those who have been through the treatment more than one year ago. Spend time researching whether the optimistic assertions can be confirmed.

What is the rationale for the treatment?

Does their explanation for the efficacy of the treatment make sense to you? If it is based upon a scientific theory, ask to see the supporting literature. If the program appears to be based upon credible basic laboratory research, contact the primary researchers directly and ask them if they believe the clinical applications of their work are reasonable and appropriate.

It may be true that sharks do not get cancer and that a component of cartilage inhibits the growth of blood vessels.[11] However, is it reasonable to take research showing a protein from shark cartilage slows the growth of blood vessels in a rabbit's eye and leap to the conclusion that it will treat cancer? Another unanswered question is whether the active substance can be absorbed when taken by mouth. It may eventually be shown that there is a benefit to a component of shark cartilage that helps in the treatment of cancer, but there is still a considerable distance to travel before I could recommend it with any confidence. On the other hand, other than the cost, it seems to carry few side effects—although I suspect the sharks might disagree.

How well documented are the cases that are used to support the treatment efficacy?

Is it reasonable to ascribe the improvement in health to the alternative treatment rather than to a concurrent medical treatment? Ideally, the positive change in a person's condition as a result of the therapy can be documented when no other confounding treatment is being received. I believe that the expectation of a therapy's success can substantially improve its efficacy by mobilizing a person's intrinsic healing response; the question regarding alternative approaches is whether there is a *specific* benefit to the particular intervention.

I suggest that my patients assessing an alternative approach ask another important question: Is it well documented that the successfully treated patients had cancer? This may seem absurd, but I have seen many patients who thought they had cancer, refused a diagnostic evaluation, followed an alternative program, and declared themselves cured.

I recently saw a delightful and very anxious woman who was convinced that the lump under her arm was metastatic breast cancer. She had been terrified to see a medical doctor so she began treatment at an alternative cancer program. First, she was encouraged to remove all the mercury amalgam fillings in her teeth. She then began a chelation therapy program designed to clear out metabolic toxins. When she came to see me, she was on at least fifteen different herbal, vitamin, and glandular supplements. I examined her and was astonished to find that her "cancer" was an infected ingrown hair that was easily treated with drainage and antibiotics!

Another patient recently contacted me before going to a five-week cancer program because a dark-field microscopy laboratory diagnosed "probable cancer." An alternative doctor had ordered the study because the man had been noticing blood after a bowel movement. He agreed to a colonoscope before treatment, which fortunately showed that his bleeding was due to hemorrhoids, not colon cancer.

Before I start to sound cynical, I want to categorically state that I believe that people with cancer do respond in exceptional ways to treatments that may not be easily explainable by current scientific understanding. The Institute of Noetic Sciences has collected more than 3,500 accounts of spontaneous remissions over the past 150 years, many following difficult-to-explain treatments ranging from krebiozen to submersion in the waters at Lourdes.[12] There is no question in my mind that people can be cured of cancer through exceptional means; the question that is relevant for someone assessing an alternative approach is: What is the likelihood that a particular treatment will be successful? To find the answers that are satisfying to you, you'll need to ask the right questions.

How long have the patients been followed since they underwent the alternative therapy?

This is important, because your choices need to be evaluated in terms of cost and benefit. This is true for any medical treatment, whether mainstream or alternative. Before agreeing to an experimental course of chemotherapy, you need to ask what are the anticipated benefits and how long will they last. If a powerful treatment causes a slight change in the size of a tumor but does not substantially influence your life expectancy, you can weigh the potential benefits against the risk and side effects. This same equation is true for alternative treatments, although the major risks are usually time and money. Ask to speak to other patients with the same type of cancer you have and find out whether the therapy offered sustained benefits. Most people who believe they were helped by an approach are happy to discuss their experiences with others facing a similar challenge. A good question to ask is: If you had to go through it again, would you take the treatment?

How much does the treatment cost?

People with cancer are often under a tremendous financial strain, which adds even more anxiety to their lives. The high cost of medical care, coupled with reduced productivity while undergoing treatments, can be a real burden to patients and their families. Therefore, it is appropriate when considering an alternative approach to ask directly, "How much is the treatment going to cost?" Of course, if it could be guaranteed that an approach provides substantial benefit I would not want to miss the opportunity because of insufficient resources. Unfortunately, most cancer treatments cannot honestly offer such a guarantee, so a cost-benefit analysis must be performed. How far will you have to travel? How long will you need to be away from work? How much does the actual treatment cost? Will you be required to purchase products to take after the formal treatment procedures? How often will you need to return for treatment? I encourage you to ask these questions so that you can integrate your hope for a successful result with the realities of day-to-day living.

What are the side effects of the treatment?

Most, but not all, alternative therapies "first do no harm." The bodywork, dietary changes, herbal medicines, and mild detoxification treatments that make up most alternative systems are usually enjoyable and without substantial risk. Programs that use intravenous agents raise a concern about infections and allergic reactions. If you are tempted to explore one of these approaches, be confident about the level of hygiene in the facility and be certain that registered nurses and physicians are in attendance.

The risk of avoiding or delaying a potentially life-saving medical treatment is number one on the list of most medical doctors' concerns regarding alternative cancer approaches. At times this can be a self-perpetuating problem, for the antagonistic attitude that some physicians express toward patients who wish to explore alternative approaches often drives them further away from potentially effective orthodox medical treatment.

A woman with breast cancer I saw several years ago is a case in point. A small calcification was discovered on her routine mammogram, leading to a needle biopsy that was positive for cancer. She was referred to a surgical oncologist, who terrified her with foreboding statistics and his recommendation for aggressive care. After seeking advice from an alternative healer, she became consciously convinced that she could cure herself without surgery, but began having recurrent fearful dreams filled with images of cancer cells invading her system. When she came to see me, she was in a state of agitated conflict over which path to take, because she had not considered that they were compatible. We developed a program that included the best of Western medicine along with holistic approaches to energize her natural immunity. Three years later she is doing well.

Remember that in the final analysis, you are responsible for your choices and your health. Your choices include your advisors as well as the therapeutic interventions you receive. Take time to question, challenge, research, and process the information you are receiving. Choose health care advisors who view you as an intelligent partner in your healing journey, recognizing that no one medical system or doctor has all the answers.

Mainstream Alternatives

Although I have been exploring alternative approaches for the past twenty-five years, I do not consider myself an expert in the alternative treatment of cancer. I have personally cared for hundreds of patients who have participated in alternative cancer programs, but I cannot say with certainty whether any specific approach has a definite impact on a person's cancer. If someone is simultaneously undergoing chemotherapy while they are changing their diet, eliminating tobacco, meditating regularly, consuming several vitamin and mineral supplements a day, taking detoxifying herbs, and seeing a homeopath, how can we know with certainty what role each component plays in improving the person's quality of life? Anecdotal reports may be fascinating and inspiring, but as the great Canadian neurologist Henry Barnett has said, "The plural of anecdote is not data."

I do believe, however, that many of the commonly available alternative medical systems can add value to the lives of people with cancer, even if they do not have a specific effect on the cancer itself. The most commonly sought out alternative doctors in the United States are chiropractors and acupuncturists. Naturopaths are gaining popularity but are currently licensed in only a few states. Homeopaths are not as commonly consulted in America but are the most popular alternative providers in Europe. Although qualified practitioners in chiropractic, acupuncture, and naturopathy complete many years of training in their disciplines, many providers expand their therapeutic repertoire beyond their original field of study. Therefore, if you are seeking their advice for the treatment of cancer, it is important that you discuss your expectations with them and see what role they are prepared to play. Because of stringent legal guidelines, most licensed alternative providers appropriately offer supportive measures rather than assume primary responsibility for people facing cancer.

Chiropractic

Although therapeutic physical manipulation was known to ancient Chinese and Greek doctors, modern chiropractic dates to David Palmer, who in 1895 manipulated a patient's spine, reportedly curing him of deafness. This led to his theory that all illness was a result of nerve impingement due to misaligned spinal vertebrae. Chiropractic, which means "done by hand," holds that adjusting the spine through physical manipulation enables nerve impulses to flow normally, restoring health to the afflicted region of the body. Because their underlying theories about health and illness are so different, medical doctors and chiropractors have been antagonists for most of the past century. After filing and winning an antitrust lawsuit against the American Medical Association in 1987, chiropractors have received somewhat greater acceptance by mainstream health care systems.

Several studies over the past decade have suggested that chiropractic can be helpful in the management of back pain, in both the acute and the chronic phases after an injury.[13, 14] Most chiropractors also receive training in nutrition and the use of food supplements, although there are different schools of thought on whether chiropractors should stay within the tradition of manipulation (straights) or expand into other areas of holistic health (mixers). I have seen many cancer patients who report that chiropractic treatments help relieve their pain. It is, of course, critical that a metastatic lesion be ruled out before an area of presumed muscle strain is treated with manipulation. There have been reported complications from cervical spine manipulation, including stroke and spinal cord injury. However, many of these complications are in people manipulated by other types of doctors, rather than by chiropractors. I have personally seen only one case of stroke, in an elderly person whose neck was manipulated by a physical therapist. Even most opponents of chiropractic admit that the risks of spinal manipulation are very small. The chiropractors that I interface with are doctors of high integrity who practice within their scope of expertise. My recommendation, if you are working with a chiropractor, is to ensure that he or she is a sensitive body worker, open to working cooperatively with your medical doctor.

Osteopathy

Osteopathy also dates its modern origin to the latter part of the eighteenth century, when Andrew Taylor Still, M.D., emphasized disease prevention and natural health enhancement. Modern osteopaths have all the privileges of medical doctors, including the ability to prescribe medications and perform surgery. In addition, they practice a selective form of manipulation designed to reestablish structural integrity. There are about forty thousand osteopathic physicians practicing in the United States today, most of them serving as primary care providers. Osteopaths are usually holistically oriented in their approach to illness and can be valuable health guides for people with cancer, helping to navigate the maze of therapeutic options.

Acupuncture

Acupuncture is the most distinguishing feature of Traditional Chinese Medicine (TCM), which also includes a vast herbal pharmacopoeia. Acupuncture became familiar to Americans after President Nixon opened diplomatic relations with China in the early seventies. The earliest Chinese medical texts date back at least three thousand years. As early as the seventeenth century, Jesuit missionaries visiting China related stories of doctors curing patients by placing needles in their skin.

As mentioned earlier, Traditional Chinese Medical doctors theorize that vital energy, called *chi*, circulates through the body within specific pathways, or *meridians*. Illness results when this life force is blocked or diminished. Despite some initial resistance, Traditional Chinese Medical practitioners have gained considerable credibility in the West and are common members of pain treatment teams. Several studies have demonstrated acupuncture's value in a variety of pain conditions, including musculoskeletal pain, migraine, and postsurgical pain.[15-17] A study in cancer patients receiving chemotherapy reported that stimulating the acupuncture point "Pericardium–6" effectively reduced nausea in over 75 percent of patients.[18] This point is located on the palm side of the wrist, about two inches above the base of the thumb. (See illustration.) It can be stimulated with a needle, with massage, or with an elastic band (Seaband) used for seasickness.

Even though we may not understand its mechanism of action in scientific terms, a system that has survived and thrived for three thousand years cannot be easily dismissed. For many people with cancer, acupuncture can be a valuable complementary treatment to relieve pain and nausea. Since acupuncture is rarely associated with side effects, other than slight discomfort at the site of needle insertion, I believe it is worth exploring if you have access to a qualified Chinese medicine practitioner.

Naturopathy

Naturopathy is a holistic health system that is currently licensed in Oregon, Washington, and Arizona. It is based upon principles that easily resonate with Ayurveda. Naturopathy describes stages of illness from optimal health to serious disease and suggests that treatment is more likely to be effective if interventions are offered before full manifestation. Diet, herbs, massage, and stress management are all important tools of naturopathic practitioners. Naturopathy presents a useful framework to integrate diverse healing modalities. I expect it to grow in popularity as more people become attracted to natural approaches for health promotion.

Homeopathy

I honestly don't understand homeopathy. Developed by Samuel Hahnemann in the early nineteenth century, homeopathy is based upon the principle that a substance or chemical that causes a symptom can be used in very diluted dosages to cure the disease that products the symptom. In other words, if castor oil causes loose stools, taking a dose of castor oil

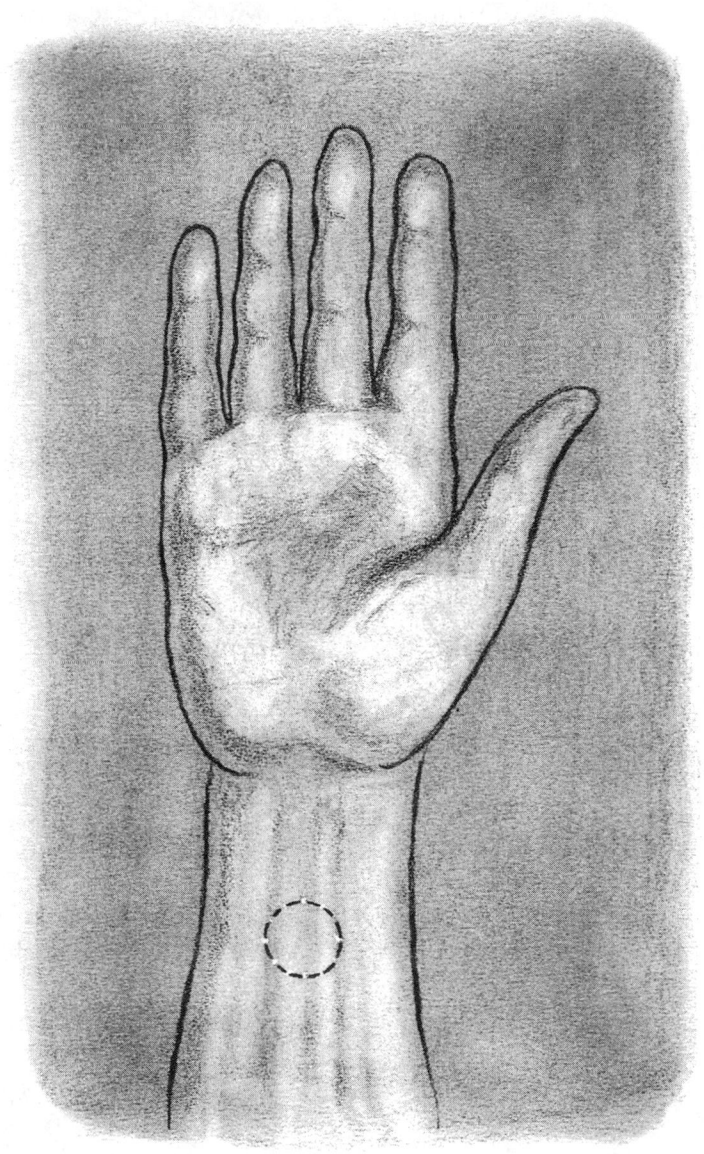

Figure 4 *Acupressure for Nausea*

that has been diluted 10^{30} times (that's one with thirty zeros after it) can cure the diarrhea of dysentery. Modern homeopathic practitioners use computerized databases to determine the correct homeopathic tincture out of almost two thousand possibilities to treat a person's complex of symptoms. According to homeopathy, the more dilute the substance, the more powerful the remedy. For many dilutions, there will not be even a single molecule of the initial substance, yet it is held, in some manner, to retain the memory of the original chemical. Because the basic tenets of homeopathy are so counterintuitive, I can understand why medical doctors have historically had trouble embracing this therapeutic approach.

However, whether we can scientifically explain homeopathy's mechanisms of action, several studies have suggested that its benefits can be verified. In people with headaches, fibromyalgia, arthritis, and allergies, homeopathic remedies have been shown to reduce symptoms, even when compared to a placebo.[19–21] A study published in the prestigious journal *Nature* raised a lot of controversy when it reported that a homeopathic dosage of an antibody caused white cells taken out of the body to release histamine, even though there was no measurable quantity of the stimulating protein—not even one molecule.[22] Although efforts to replicate these findings were unsuccessful, this study opened a crack in our solid material view of cause and effect. Orthodox medicine recognizes that *less* can sometimes be *more*, as in studies that have shown that lower doses of aspirin may be more effective than higher ones in the prevention of stroke, but it has not yet come up with a cogent explanation of how *none* can be better than *some*.

Even though I admit that I don't understand homeopathy, there are several aspects of this system that are appealing to me. First, it is completely safe, for even potentially toxic substances are diluted beyond detectable levels. Second, homeopathy recognizes, as did Jivaka in the Ayurvedic tradition, that almost everything in the world can have therapeutic value—this includes herbs, minerals, insects, and animals. Finally, I actually like the fact that at this time we cannot understand its mechanism of action from a scientific perspective. It reminds me that our concept of "truth" is very much based upon an agreed-upon perspective that changes over time. It's conceivable to me that at some future point we may understand that a substance can exert a field effect that extends beyond any direct molecular interactions in a way analogous to the way a small undetected outer planet can alter the orbit of Mars. Time will tell whether homeopathy and the questions it raises will be relegated to the footnotes of history or be seen as an opening to a new paradigm. If you have cancer and access to a qualified homeopath, it is probably among the safest alternative approaches to enliven your internal healing force.

Responsive and Responsible Healing

I believe that people facing cancer can become true experts in their illness. An expert is someone who knows what is known and acknowledges what is unknown. No one is as dedicated to your well being as you are. Therefore, in your journey to wholeness, you must be the captain of your vessel. Seek information that is empowering to you, recognizing that your individual situation is unique. Maintain an attitude of flexibility and keep your heart and mind open to possibilities.

Any therapeutic approach can be beneficial as a focal point to mobilize your healing energy. Whether it is a medication, herb, vitamin, homeopathic tincture, or affirmation, the intervention will be useful if you are open to its healing power. Every doctor has seen patients who fail to gain the predicted benefit of a treatment and others whose response far exceeds expectations. This is why it is important that you do your homework before proceeding with a therapy. The more confident you are in the intervention and the health provider with whom you are working, the more you will be able to align your inner doctor with your outer one.

On the other hand, resist the impulse to surrender all your power to an outside authority, be it an orthodox or an alternative doctor. It is natural when we are sick to want a benign all-knowing parental figure to take care of us, and good doctors will assume their rightful role as nurturing guides. We need to remember that doctors are playing a time-honored role, but in this information age that role is changing. In addition to being a compassionate caregiver, the doctor needs to be someone who educates and empowers. Don't be afraid to ask your doctor tough questions, such as, "If you or a family member were facing my situation, would you proceed with this intervention?" Ask how long you should expect to wait until you see an effect. If you decide to explore a particular approach, determine a reasonable period of time to assess its effectiveness. This is as true for an experimental medical treatment as it is for an alternative therapy. Tell your health advisors that you want them to be honest, particularly if they are not convinced they have anything more to offer you.

Make your commitments, but try not to be too dogmatic. If you find yourself being emotionally activated by someone challenging your choices, remember the sage words of the German novelist and philosopher Thomas Mann, who said, "We are most likely to get angry and excited in our opposition to some idea when we are ourselves are not quite certain of our own position and are inwardly tempted to take the other side."

Remember that healing is different from curing. Even if a particular herb, enzyme, or homeopathic remedy does not produce the specific desired effect, if you are learning about yourself and discovering the deeper meaning of life, you are on a healing path. Ultimately, it is being awake on the journey that will return you to wholeness.

Commitment to Wholeness

Our bodies are the end products of our experiences and interpretations. To change our bodies, we need to change our experiences. Make a commitment to change your life in the direction of greater love and caring for yourself and those close to you.

1. I commit to my role as the primary healer in my life, using doctors and health practitioners as allies and guides.

2. I commit to assessing alternative medical modalities with both my heart and my mind, exploring those approaches that resonate with my nature and seem reasonable to me.

3. I commit to taking responsibility for my body and my choices. If a recommendation offered feels appropriate for my condition, I will pursue it. If the suggestion does not seem suitable for me, before proceeding with the advice of a health advisor I will ask elucidating questions until my concerns are satisfied.

CHAPTER 14

Holistically Specific

Approaching Common Cancers
from a Mind-Body Perspective

There is no difficulty that enough love will not conquer; no disease that
enough love will not heal.—EMMET FOX, *THE SERMON ON THE MOUNT*

Many of the holistic approaches that are useful for people facing cancer
are helpful regardless of what type of cancer they may be facing. In truth,
these approaches, which ultimately serve to remind us of our state of
wholeness, are valuable whether or not we are facing a life-threatening
illness. I am aware that my life in this body will eventually come to a
close. Although our youth-focused culture diligently tries to push mortality out of our conscious awareness, we are all coping with a terminal
process if we identify ourselves with our physical body and its inevitable
limitations in time. This is why I so strongly encourage the regular experience of deeper levels of silence within our awareness through meditation, because it allows us to glimpse an aspect of our nature that is
beyond time and space—beyond boundaries. From boundaries arises
separation, and in the possibility of separation, fear is born. I think it's
safe to say that all suffering stems from our fear of separation. It may be
the fear of separating from our material possessions, our loved ones, or
our bodies. In every case, fear is the antithesis of wholeness, and therefore, the remedy for fear is the infusion of spirit, which is unbounded
and unconditional in its essential nature. Reestablishing our connection
with the unbounded and indivisible ocean within is the essence of true
healing.

On the other hand, I realize that when we are facing an urgent, real-life challenge, simply hearing that we are ultimately spiritual rather than physical beings may not provide a tangible enough life raft to bring comfort or relief. In the midst of desperation, being reminded that there is a quiet, stable inner core sounds good, but unless we can access it directly, it may seem more like a mirage than a real oasis in the desert. This is when the technologies of mind-body medicine become important. Daily meditation, a diet rich in life-promoting foods, a daily routine that allows us to harmonize with natural rhythms, consciously seeking sensory nourishment, openly and honestly expressing our emotions, loving supportive relationships—these all help create a personal environment that allows us to settle into a state of greater comfort and knowingness. In this return to our innate wholeness, anxiety and fear subside and our natural healing forces are enlivened.

Although these general health-promoting mind-body approaches are very powerful, people facing cancer inevitably want to know what specifically they can do for their illness. In addition to general health-promoting practices, people seek out interventions that address the individual aspects of their concerns as well as their underlying universality. "What foods should I eat for my prostate cancer?" "Is there a specific herb I can take for my type of lymphoma?" "What visualization should I use for my metastatic lung cancer?" These are the questions I hear every day from my patients. When I see people in follow-up sessions, I am no longer surprised at how often people have difficulty finding the time to meditate, prepare a healthy meal, or go for a walk in the woods, but are regularly taking their blue-green algae and shark cartilage several times per day. I think we may all have a basic need to latch on to some tangible solutions before we are able to appreciate more expanded approaches, yet I believe symptom-oriented interventions alone cannot catalyze the necessary transformation in consciousness that is at the basis of true healing.

Most Western cancer treatment protocols are very specific. The treatment for breast cancer is different from the treatment for leukemia. The interventions for localized breast cancer are distinct from those for metastatic disease. This level of specificity is not possible, nor even necessarily desirable, when exploring approaches derived from a mind-body medicine perspective. The basis of mind-body medicine is focusing attention on the person who has the disease rather than on the disease that has the person. And yet, out of the full repertoire of mind-body approaches, we can emphasize specific interventions that may be particularly helpful for different types of cancers. Different classes of malignancies seem to carry their own constellation of issues and concerns that, when addressed, can improve quality of life and offer profound opportunities for emotional and spiritual healing.

In this chapter I will address the role of mind-body interventions in three of the most common cancers afflicting our Western society—breast, prostate, and colon. The holistic approach to these three cancers can be used as models for similar malignancies. For example, the recommendations outlined for breast cancer can be applied to other tumors of the female reproductive system, including ovarian, uterine, and cervical cancers. The approaches for prostate cancer are also relevant for testicular cancer. The discussion of mind-body approaches for colon cancer can also be useful for other digestive tract malignancies, including tumors of the stomach, pancreas, and liver. Please remember that these more specific suggestions are in no way to be considered a substitute for appropriate medical care. Rather, they are offered as a way to help you focus your healing energies as effectively as possible.

Breast Cancer—The Shadow in the Nurturer

Hope springs eternal in the human breast.

ALEXANDER POPE

Elizabeth did not consider herself to be a vain woman. With the support of her family, she navigated her way through the trials and challenges of her breast cancer therapy. Her friends marveled at how even-tempered she had been when she received the initial news of her diagnosis. After rationally reviewing her treatment options with her surgeon, she decided that a simple mastectomy with postoperative radiation would provide her the best chance for a good outcome.

It wasn't until a month after she had completed her treatments that she began feeling that getting out of bed in the morning was a major task. She found herself getting anxious at the thought of taking a shower and avoided looking at her body in the mirror at all costs. Fortunately, with the help of a therapist, a cancer support group, and a meditation and yoga class, she gradually worked through her pain. She was then able to develop a new relationship with her body that acknowledged both her grief for her loss as well as appreciation for its genuine beauty and support.

The breast is a tissue rich with symbolism. As newborn infants we quickly learn to associate the warmth, softness, and sweet smell of mother with the delicious nectar that nourishes our body and soul. The glandular mounds that arise in the pubescent girl are the most obvious anatomical identifiers that distinguish human females from their male counterparts. Our mammary glands remind us of our biological inheritance as mammals. The human breast may be the primordial mandala that promises us the ultimate rewards when we reach the center of the symbol. Considering the powerful associations we have with the breast, it is not surprising how cancer in this tissue creates such deep physical, emotional, and spiritual distress.

As a man, I cannot pretend to fully appreciate the significance of having cancer of the breast. Although almost 1,500 men will develop breast cancer this year in the United States, this number pales in comparison to the 180,000 American women annually diagnosed with breast cancer. It is by far the most common malignant tumor that women face, and it is estimated that almost one in eight women will develop breast cancer during their lifetimes. This is about twice the incidence of breast cancer experienced sixty years ago. By comparison, lung cancer in women is a distant second, with less than half as many cases diagnosed yearly, although more women die from lung cancer each year than from breast cancer. At least in part due to early diagnosis and improved treatment protocols, the mortality rate from breast cancer has fallen over the past several years, despite a rise in its overall occurrence.[1]

We do not know the cause of breast cancer. Although there is an increased risk of a daughter's developing breast cancer if her mother or sister was affected, genetics seems to play a relatively minor role. Although other factors such as how old a woman was when she started her menstrual periods, first became pregnant, and began menopause play some role, more than half the time no identifiable risk factors can be identified. This lack of understanding continues to motivate the search for other causes that may account for the rising incidence of this illness.

The suspicion that there must be modifiable risk factors for breast cancer comes from studies that show a wide variation in the incidence of this disease around the world. The rate of breast cancer in the United States and Europe is four to seven times higher than in China and Japan. Although you may think that this suggests this illness favors certain racial or ethnic groups more than others, this doesn't seem to be the case. If you look at Asian women who migrate to the West, their risk of breast cancer rises the longer they're here. Asian American women born in the United

States have rates of breast cancer almost equal to those of Caucasian Americans.[2] Most cancer scientists now agree that environmental and lifestyle choices must play a significant role in the high rates of breast cancer in the West.

Diet and Breast Cancer

If there are factors that we can influence through our choices, what are they? Nutrition is the area that receives the most attention, and although there are many positive signs, we don't yet know how effective nutritional approaches can be in the prevention and treatment of breast cancer. As discussed generally in chapter 3 on nutrition, there is a fairly strong linkage between dietary animal fat and breast cancer. In societies where people eat more animal foods, there is more breast cancer. There are two basic theories as to why this may be. We know that diets high in saturated fats can alter the fatty composition of cell membranes and may reduce the potency of immune system cells.[3] Dietary fat is also associated with higher levels of circulating estrogen, which may contribute to the development of breast cancer.[4] However, the relationship between fat and breast cancer is not that simple. We know that high-fat diets are associated with obesity. It turns out that being overweight may actually slightly *decrease* the risk of breast cancer in women who are in their reproductive years, but *increase* the risk in women who have been through menopause. Although its degree of importance continues to be debated, I believe it's safe to say that reducing your intake of animal fat can be beneficial if you are facing breast cancer.

The other side of the dietary fat issue is the role of fiber in breast cancer. Many studies from around the world have shown that fewer women develop breast cancer in cultures whose diets are rich in fiber. Because fruits, vegetables, and whole grains are the richest sources of fiber, people who have diets high in fiber also tend to have a lower intake of animal fat. Both premenopausal and postmenopausal vegetarian women tend to have lower levels of circulating estrogen, possibly because the plant fiber prevents the reabsorption of estrogen that has been released in their bile.

Importantly, certain types of plant foods seem to have specific protective effects. The fiber, along with other chemical ingredients, in soybeans seems to have unique health-enhancing benefits on breast cancer. Clues from both laboratory studies and clinical research suggest that the class of phytochemicals known as isoflavonoids may be converted into natural forms of estrogens that can block the tendency of breast tissue to undergo malignant changes. Natural chemicals found in soybeans added to breast cancer cells in a petri dish inhibit their growth, but it's unclear whether we can achieve similar levels of isoflavonoids shown to be effective in these laboratory studies simply from eating more soybean-derived foods.[5] Similar studies in animals have shown that mice with breast cancers fed a high-soy diet show fewer metastases than their sisters who do not receive the soybean phytochemicals. Women in China and Japan consume much higher quantities of soy foods than American women, which may be one of the important reasons why they have less than 20 percent of the breast cancer we have here in the United States.

Another potentially useful natural breast-cancer-fighting chemical is found in cauliflower. This substance, known as a carbinol, may also act to block the cancer-causing effects of estrogens on breast cells. Many environmentalists fear that synthetic chemicals in our air, water, and soil mimic our natural hormones, provoking the formation of cancer. It has been suggested that natural plant chemicals found in soy products and vegetables may help to inactivate or block the effects of these toxic endocrine disruptors on our tissues.

If you are facing breast cancer, my bottom-line recommendation regarding nutrition is to substantially reduce your intake of animal fat and supplement your vegetable and whole grain diet with soybean-derived foods such as tofu, tempeh, and soy milk. In addition to getting more of these important healing phytochemicals, this diet is rich in antioxidant vitamins and the high fiber will help to regulate your bowels.

Vitamins and Breast Cancer

Does it make sense to supplement with vitamins if you are facing breast cancer? Over the years, a number of reports have suggested that beta-carotene and vitamins A, C, and E may have a protective effect in breast cancer. Of these antioxidant nutrients, beta-carotene and vitamin A have shown the most consistent benefit, but these effects have been modest. Taking supplementary vitamins has not demonstrated as clear a benefit as eating a diet that is naturally rich in antioxidant vitamins. It seems that Nature has packaged her healing chemicals in the forms that are most nurturing—fresh fruits and vegetables rather than tablets and capsules.

Another natural biochemical called coenzyme Q has been reported to help some women with breast cancer. This compound plays an important role in our cells' energy production, and a deficiency of this chemical has been implicated in contributing to DNA damage. Although some call this substance *vitamin* Q10, it cannot legitimately be classified as a vitamin for unlike a vitamin, we are fully capable of synthesizing it through our own metabolic processes. Recent reports have suggested that it may have antioxidant activity, reminding us again that many natural substances can provide healing benefits through many different mechanisms. An oncologist and his research group from Denmark gave 390 milligrams a day of coenzyme Q to thirty-two women and reported improvement in six.[6] They later described three more women with rather dramatic improvements that the researchers attributed to coenzyme Q.[7] Unfortunately, after their initial encouraging results, very little additional research has been conducted. Interestingly, despite this rather limited scientific evidence, you can now buy coenzyme Q in almost every health food store. To date, I have not seen any reports of toxicity from this substance.

As I suggested in chapter 4, I think that it is reasonable to supplement with a good antioxidant multivitamin while you are receiving chemotherapy or radiation treatments, particularly if your appetite is suppressed and you are finding it difficult to eat a balanced diet. Over the longer term, I believe it's prudent to supplement your diet with additional beta-carotene, aiming for a daily intake of about 25,000 International Units. Although you can take it as a vitamin supplement, one of the best ways to ensure that you are receiving adequate dosages of this important antioxidant is by drinking some freshly prepared carrot juice on a daily basis. Eight ounces provides about 15,000 IU, so two cups a day will be plenty. Although you may see a slight orange tinge to your skin, beta-carotene is nontoxic and is converted to vitamin A as needed. At this time I don't think there is enough evidence to be aggressive about pushing vitamins E or C, but you should be receiving adequate amounts if you are following a balanced low-fat, high-fiber diet.

Body Awareness

When our bodies are ill, we often withdraw our attention deeper into our minds. Being conscious of our physical states is sometimes simply too uncomfortable, so we attempt to divert our attention to something in the past or future. I commonly see women with breast cancer who put up a psychological and emotional barrier between their conscious awareness and their bodies. They avoid looking at and touching their bodies and are even more uncomfortable allowing a loved one to see their physical vulnerability. This type of psychological avoidance after surgery may initially be a natural and healthy response, allowing some time for physical and emotional healing. But at some point, learning to see, feel, and love the body after it has undergone a physical transformation is essential to the healing process.

Loving Touch. The most direct way we have of showing affection and appreciation is to lovingly touch the object of our love. As soon as you feel ready, I encourage you to begin caressing your chest and breast area around the site of your wound. If you have had a lumpectomy or mastectomy, begin with the arm on the affected side. Make certain your hands are washed and warm, and start by gently massaging each of your fingers, moving from the tips to the wrist. Then in a slow milking manner, massage your forearm, compressing your muscles around the entire arm. At the elbow, use a circular and gentle pinching motion. Continue to compress the muscles in your upper arm, moving repetitively from your elbow to your shoulder. Massage over your shoulder in a circular fashion, gently squeezing as you move along the upper bundle of muscle fibers between your shoulder blade and neck. Very gently massage the area below your clavicle, repeatedly moving from your shoulder to your breastbone. Now very lightly massage in a circular motion around the site of your surgery. Have the intention in your awareness to send healing, compassionate, loving energy to the tissues that have been challenged by your illness and the treatments for the illness. If the wound has completely closed, try using a light massage oil such as almond, olive, or jojoba to which you have added a few drops of vitamin E. In addition to enhancing healing and reducing discomfort, a daily massage can help relieve swelling due to disruption in the lymphatic drainage from the tumor, surgery, or radiation.

Perform this massage on a daily basis, and when you are comfortable, do so while watching yourself in the mirror. If you do this procedure prior to a bath or shower, allow the oil to soak in for a few minutes before washing with a light soap. If strong emotions rise to the surface, allow them to flow as you grieve your loss, while simultaneously expressing your appreciation for the recovery process.

According to Ayurveda and Traditional Chinese Medicine (TCM), we have a number of vital points on the surface of our body that can be stimulated to enhance our healing forces. Known as marma points in Ayurveda and meridian points in TCM, these specific sites are considered to be the junction points between consciousness and matter. Gentle massage of these spots has been traditionally used to enliven the life force

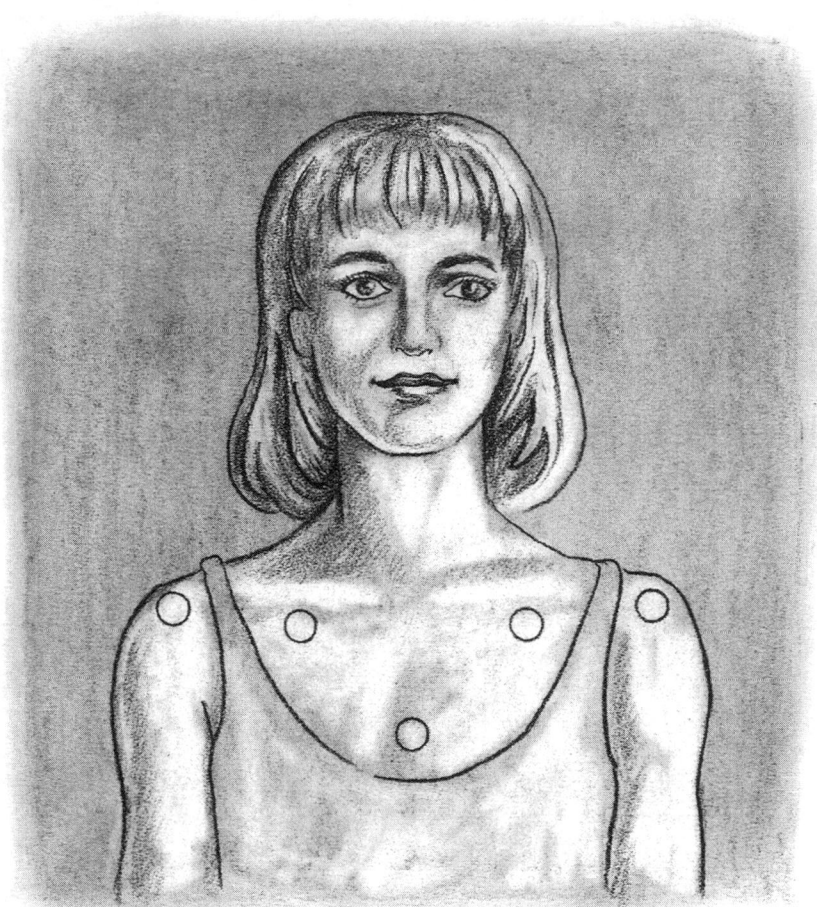

Figure 5 **Marma Points**

when it is blocked. Try gently massaging an area right below the midpoint of the clavicles and another point at the outer end of the clavicles where they join with the shoulders. Rubbing with a gentle circular motion for a couple of minutes is said to help enliven the pran, or life force, in the chest area. One of the major vital points known as Hridaya or "heart" marma is located over the center of the sternum. Applying a diluted aromatic essential oil will provide a mild chemical stimulation to this vital point. Try rubbing in a few drops of basil, clary sage, juniper, peppermint, or thyme oil after a warm shower and enjoy the soothing stimulation these natural oils offer.

Gentle Stretching. After surgery and radiation, it is common for the surrounding tissues to tighten and stiffen. When this occurs, it is easy to fall
into a negative cycle in which the discomfort of the shortened tissues re-
stricts movement, creating more discomfort. As soon as your surgeon
tells you it is safe, begin very gentle stretching exercises to expand your
chest muscles. These should be performed with conscious breathing
awareness and sensitivity for your body.

I recommend the following three stretches. In the first exercise, place
your fists together about four inches in front of your sternum with your
arms parallel to the ground. With a slow deep inhalation, gently pull your
elbows backwards, holding for a few moments and then returning your fists
to the front with your exhalation. Repeat this three times, stretching to a
position of comfortable tension but not to the point of discomfort.

In the second exercise, clasp your fingers together in front of your
sternum and with a deep slow inhalation, raise both arms in front of you
over your head. Hold the stretch for a few seconds and then return your
hands to their original position. Repeat this exercise three to five times.

In the third exercise, begin with your hands over your upper belly
and, with a deep breath, roll your hands outwards toward your sides as
you bring your elbows back as if trying to touch them together. Gently
perform this stretch a few times, returning your hands to the front with
each exhalation.

The best time to perform these stretches is when your muscles are
warm. They can be done for few minutes while in the shower. Be certain to
do them with awareness and sensitivity. Go to the point of a comfortable
tension, but do not overdo them, for excessive stretching will increase tension rather than the flexibility you are seeking. Breathe deeply throughout
these exercises, and you will feel improved energy and vitality in your chest.

Emotional Healing

Dealing with a life-threatening illness is undeniably painful. Considering
how upset human beings can get over the little things in life—a minor automobile accident, a large-than-expected tax bill, an insensitive comment
from a friend—it is fully understandable that waves of painful emotions
arise as you face the most serious challenge of your life. Allow yourself
the freedom and the time to experience your emotions without the continuous need to be a brave soldier. Like a physical boil, emotional wounds
need to release what is being retained in order for deep healing to occur.

There is no one right way to process the emotional grief and pain associated with illness. Some people find they benefit from spending some time alone in nature, while others find that constant human companionship provides the support they need. Feeling somewhat emotionally isolated from your family and friends is a common reaction when you first learn of your illness. Studies have shown that women who participate in support groups feel better and live longer. I strongly encourage you to communicate your fears and hopes to loving family and friends and engage their support in your healing journey. Feel your feelings, express your feelings, and write about your feelings while at the same time seeking to connect with the underlying quiet ocean within you that is beyond the waves of emotions that are disturbing your peace. Seek the deeper meaning and the opportunity for spiritual growth inherent in every crisis, and have faith that life is always propelling us on an evolutionary journey.

If you feel overwhelmed by sadness, be certain to communicate with your health care providers and be open to receiving temporary pharmaceutical help to get you over the rough spots. Many of the new selective serotonin reuptake inhibitor (SSRI) antidepressants are very effective with relatively few side effects and can help to boost your brain's natural mood-elevating chemicals. Saint-John's-wort (*Hypericum perforatum*), an herb well known to ancient medical herbalists, has been shown in several studies to be an effective antidepressant for mild to moderate symptoms. The usual recommended dosage is 300 milligrams three times a day. There are very few reported side effects from this herb, although it may take a month or longer to see a benefit. Although hypericum causes the skin of certain animals to become sensitive to sunlight, this effect has not been seen in people. In Germany, where herbal approaches are increasingly embraced by the mainstream medical system, more doses of Saint-John's-wort are prescribed each year than all the pharmaceutical antidepressant medications combined. Saint-John's-wort is a gift from nature, which can be a useful ingredient of a holistic healing program.

Nurturing the Nurturer

Most women have received messages from an early age that at least part of their role in life is to care for others. As mothers, sisters, daughters, wives, and lovers, women give of themselves, at times to the point of depletion. If you recognize that you are a person who is capable of exhausting yourself as you give to others, I appeal to you to take time for yourself while you are recovering from your cancer. Be as willing to receive love and support as you are to provide it for others. If even with a serious illness you have difficulty asking for help, consider that you will be of much greater service to others if you are willing to nurture yourself. It is impossible for an empty well to quench anyone's thirst. Open your heart to the healing spirit that exists within yourself and in those who love you, and you will be in good company as you travel along your path to wholeness.

Prostate Cancer—Restricting the Flow

The longest part of the journey is said to be the passing of the gate.
MARCUS TERENTIUS VARRO

Sam Spiegel took pride in how fit he looked and felt at age fifty-five. He had stopped smoking years ago, worked out regularly at his fitness club, and recently changed his diet. Fortunately, with his successes in business, Sam was not excessively burdened by ongoing spousal support to his two ex-wives. He was confident when he went for his annual medical checkup that he would receive a clean bill of health. Consequently, he was very distressed when his physician told him that he felt a small nodule on his prostate gland. Although Sam's first impulse was to ignore his doctor's advice to have a biopsy, his borderline PSA level convinced him to see a urologist. The biopsy showed an early localized and treatable cancer.

As Sam progressed through the treatment journey, he searched for the meaning of his illness. He looked not only at the message his cancer was sending, but wondered why it had arisen in his prostate. In his meditations and dreams, Sam began to see his prostate cancer as a metaphor for his use of masculine energy. He discovered patterns in his personal and work relationships that suggested obstacles in his ability to express his energy and creativity in ways that were mutually nurturing. His healing journey was occurring on physical, emotional, and spiritual levels.

What can you say about a condition that ultimately develops in over two-thirds of men if they live to age eighty? This is what studies of men who have died from other causes tell us about prostate cancer. In the majority of these cases the cancer was only detected under a microscope (called histologic or latent cancer) and seldom caused clinical problems. Still, prostate cancer is now the most frequently diagnosed malignancy in the United States, with over 300,000 cases diagnosed this year.

It is not nearly as common a cancer in other parts of the world. The rate of clinically apparent prostate cancer in African American men is 25 times higher than in Japanese men and 120 times greater than the incidence in Chinese men from Shanghai![8] A high level of male hormones is an important risk factor in prostate cancer, but this alone does not tell the entire story. Although the rates of latent prostate cancer may be similar around the world, there are great differences in how rapidly a microscopic cancer grows to the point at which it is detectable.

The prostate gland is the only organ in the body that continues to grow throughout life. The prostate of a man at sixty-five years of age is two or three times larger than it was when he was twenty years old. The prostate normally releases proteins, enzymes, metals, and other substances to help sperm move efficiently, but why it should continue to enlarge long after a man is likely to father a child is a mystery. We do know that prostate cancer goes through many steps before it expresses itself as a medical problem. In the early stage, genetic mutations occur that lead to a limited number of cancerous prostate cells. These may never cause any harm and may be discovered only incidentally during an autopsy. In a certain percentage of men, the tumor grows so that prostate cancer can be diagnosed through an examination or an elevation in the prostate specific antigen (PSA) level. If there are further genetic changes, the prostate cancer cells may break free of the prostate and travel to other sites in the body, usually involving the lymph nodes and the bone. This entire process may take years to progress, and a small localized prostate cancer may never cause life-threatening problems.

Depending upon the stage of cancer, standard medical treatments can vary from cautious monitoring to hormonal therapy, surgery, radiation, and chemotherapy. With growing awareness of this common cancer, more men are being diagnosed at earlier stages of disease. The best treatment for early localized prostate disease is debated, considering that the cancer may grow only slowly over years although prostate cancer in young men tends to be more aggressive. On the other end of the spectrum, metastatic prostate cancer is a serious and life-threatening problem, usually requiring chemotherapy and hormonal therapy to control the illness.

Hormones, Diet, and the Prostate

We know that prostate cancer is sensitive to male hormones. Studies from cultures where eunuchs exist have shown that men who cannot produce male hormones rarely get prostate cancer. Hormonal manipulation is an important form of treatment in men who have prostate cancer, although not all cancer cells remain sensitive to male hormones throughout the course of the disease. Recognizing that clinical prostate cancer rates vary widely throughout the world and that male hormones have a provocative effect, researchers have looked at factors that may explain the vast differences between cultures. Once again, diet seems to play an important role.

Like breast cancer, rates of prostate cancer are highest in societies where animal fat is a major part of the diet. If you follow Japanese men as they migrate from their native homeland to the United States, their risk of prostate cancer gradually approaches that of their host country, presumably because they begin to follow a more typical American lifestyle and diet. We don't really understand how dietary fat influences prostate cancer, but it is suspected that it alters the production of sex hormones. In an interesting study comparing male hormone levels in American and South African black men, it was shown that South African men fed an American diet showed increases in their testosterone levels, whereas black North American men fed a predominantly vegetarian diet showed the opposite effect.[9]

The story gets more interesting. As I mentioned earlier, Chinese men have among the lowest incidence of prostate cancer in the world. And of course, soy products, which are rich in phytoestrogens, comprise a large part of their daily diet. In fact, it has been suggested that the typical person living in China consumes thirty-five times the soy products of an average American. A group of researchers from Europe and China looked at the prostate fluid of healthy Chinese, English, and Portuguese men and found substantially elevated levels of certain natural phytoestrogens in Chinese men compared to the Europeans.[10] The suggestion, once again, is that natural substances in soy products and vegetables have a protective effect against cancer.

Does a diet rich in phytoestrogens help someone who already has prostate cancer? It is definitely too soon to make such a claim, although a recent report from Australia provides some hope that there may be value to adding phytoestrogens to your diet. In this publication, a sixty-six-year-old man with prostate cancer took 160 milligrams per day of phytoestrogens for a week before his prostate surgery. When his surgeons operated on him, they found that many of the cancerous cells had died, a response that is usually seen only after high doses of estrogen drugs.[11]

As is often true in nature, things are not as simple as we might wish them to be. Recent studies looking at the relationship between fat and prostate cancer have discovered that a component of fat called alpha-linolenic acid may be the portion associated with an increased risk.[12] Although most dietary alpha-linolenic acid comes from red meat and butter, flaxseed, canola, and soybean oils are botanical sources. Alpha-linolenic acid comprises 50 percent of flaxseed oil, 12 percent of canola oil, and about 7 percent of soybean oil.

What should we do with this information? Since there is essentially no risk, I would encourage you to reduce your total intake of dietary fat and favor fruits, vegetables, and grains. The phytoestrogens found in soy products seem to be the most beneficial, although other phytochemicals present in lentils, oat bran, garlic, squash, pears, and plums may also be important. What about potential concerns over the fatty acid found in soy and flaxseed oil? I think this information highlights the risk of trying to focus on only one component of a natural product. It may eventually be confirmed that alpha-linolenic acid has a stimulating effect on prostate cancer, but I suspect it will be shown that the other benefits of phytoestrogen-rich foods far outweigh the effect of a single fatty acid representing only 7 percent of the oil of the soybean. The amount of alpha-linolenic acid in a standard helping of tofu is less than one-third of 1 percent of our recommended daily total dietary fat. Until more complete information is available, I do not advocate adding flaxseed oil to your diet, but I do favor soy-derived products such as tofu, tempeh, and textured vegetable protein.

Is it worth supplementing with vitamins or minerals? At various times vitamins A, C, E, and D have been suggested to offer some protection against prostate cancer, although the benefits have been neither overwhelming nor consistent. One of the most promising nutritional substances that may be helpful in prostate cancer is lycopene, a carotenoid that does not get converted into vitamin A. Tomatoes are the major source of this powerful antioxidant, which seems to have a propensity for concentrating in the prostate gland. In several studies, men who have a high intake of tomatoes in their diet have a substantially lower risk of prostate cancer.[13, 14] Your tomatoes can be consumed fresh, as soup, as juice, or in the form of a sauce. Even regular pizza eaters seem to benefit! Unless you are allergic to tomatoes, I encourage you to eat lots of them along with your other vegetables, fruits, whole grains, and beans.

Body Awareness

As with any illness, men with prostate cancer have a tendency to withdraw their attention from the area of difficulty. Considering the emotional charge associated with our reproductive organs, it is not surprising that some men want to downplay the significance of this common cancer. Yet I have found that men with prostate cancer who are willing to focus their attention on their bodies often feel more positive and less fearful about their lives and their health.

In addition to a daily oil massage, I encourage men with prostate cancer to perform a perineal massage with warm almond or olive oil. Apply the oil in a stroking motion along the inner sides of your thighs and in the area between your anus and your scrotum. Afterwards, take a warm sitz bath and practice tightening and releasing your anal sphincter muscle, using a procedure often recommended for pregnant women, known as Kegels or pelvic toners. In the yoga tradition, this exercise is called the "root lock."

To perform pelvic toners, sit comfortably, lengthen the spine upward, and lift your chest. Using a contracting and lifting motion, draw the perineum upward and inward. Feel the anus and buttocks contract as well as lift, but keep the rest of the body relaxed. Hold this pose for five deep breaths, relax the pelvic floor muscles, and then repeat the process. This exercise helps to tone the pelvic musculature and enliven the flow of energy into this area.

The following two pelvis opening and stretching exercises can also be helpful in improving energy flow, particularly as you are recovering from surgery or radiation. Be certain to discuss with your urologist when it is safe to perform these postures, and always do them with sensitivity and awareness.

1. Butterfly pose. Sit comfortably on a firm padded surface with your spine erect. Place the soles of both feet in front of you with your knees bent and together. Gently spread your legs so you are feeling gentle ten-

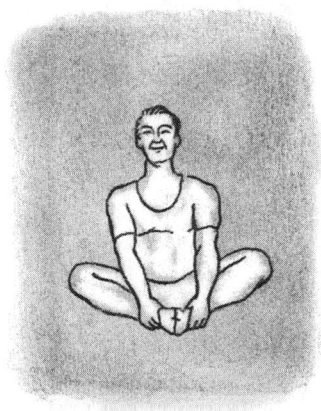

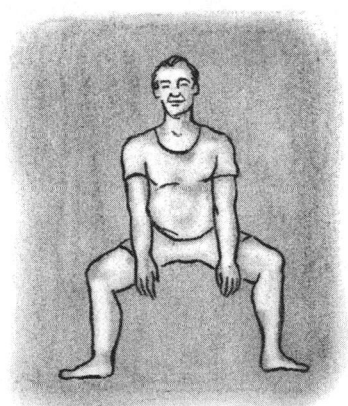

BUTTERFLY POSE HORSE STANCE

Figure 6 **Yoga Postures**

sion in your groin. Hold this position for a few moments, breathing easily into the tension, then return to the resting position. Be very careful not to go beyond the point of a comfortable stretch.

2. Horse stance. Stand with your legs about two shoulder widths apart with your toes pointing outward. Supporting your weight with your hands on your thighs, slowly and carefully bend your knees until you feel a gentle stretch. Again, hold this position for a few breaths, then return to an upright position.

Emotions and Masculinity

Although it may be a cliché, I believe it's true that men are not as comfortable exploring or expressing their emotions as women. I suspect that both by nature and nurture men tend to deal with their fears and anxieties through activity rather than through emotional processing and expression. And yet, the emotional pain of confronting our mortality is real and provides a powerful opportunity for healing and wisdom.

I encourage you to look for the meaning in your prostate cancer. The most important risk factor for this illness is being a man. Since male hormones provoke prostate cancer, there is some validity to the suggestion that the more we are driven by our male energy, the more we are at risk for prostate cancer. Like Sam, described at the beginning of this chapter, it is not uncommon for men with prostate cancer to have been very successful in the world, but to have had ongoing difficulties in their personal relationships. The powerful warrior drives in men often compete with our softer, nurturing forces. The male energy, whether we are man or woman, is inherently goal-oriented and continuously on a quest for accomplishment. The female energy, whether we are man or woman, is governed by seasons, cycles, and rhythms. It is inherently self-referential, intuitive, and nonlinear. A complete human being, whether we are man or woman, can travel in either realm and experience the rewards of both sides of our natures.

Facing a serious illness affords us the opportunity to explore and awaken aspects of our natures that may have been previously dormant. If you are facing prostate cancer, I encourage you to look inside yourself and ask what more you need to feel fulfilled. Evaluate your relationships and heal those that need attention. Look at those things you have always wanted to do but have been putting off for years, or perhaps your whole life, because of pressing responsibilities and deadlines. For all the anguish that cancer brings, it carries a hidden gift, which is to remind us that every moment is precious. If there ever was a good time to heal wounds from the past or live out a lifelong dream, this is it! I encourage you to take advantage of this opportunity to deepen your connectedness to the eternal wisdom of life, which is quietly calling us to remember who we really are.

Cancer and Sexuality

Our bodies are sources of pleasure and pain. When we are experiencing physical distress, any new bodily sensation or movement may be anticipated with trepidation. Cancer extacts a substantial toll from the body, and the thought of receiving sexual pleasure when you are hurting may seem remote or even repugnant. In addition to physical discomfort, there are other components of the cancer process that can influence our sexuality. Body image is often affected due to hair loss from treatments, changes in weight, scars from operations, and alterations in hormonal levels. Particularly if the cancer has affected a sexual organ, the prospect of physical intimacy may be intimidating. And yet, sexual energy is the essence of the life force and, when the time is appropriate, can be an important component of the healing process.

I encourage you to love your body *because of*, not *in spite of*, what it has gone through. Throughout your healing journey, attend to your body with love and compassion. Send it thoughts of appreciation for tolerating the difficult therapies required. On a daily basis, sensitively caress your body as a source of pleasure. As you are recovering from your treatments, gently explore the sensations around the treated areas, discovering the boundaries between comfort and discomfort. As your healing progresses, notice the shift toward greater ease in your body and the expansion of pleasurable sensations.

Remember that you can make love without having sex. When you are ready to share physical intimacy with your cherished one, approach each other as spiritual beings, using your bodies to express love. Create a sacred space, attending to the sights, sounds, and aromas in your environment. Touch with sensitivity and subtlety, providing feedback on what is comfortable and what is not. Play with the energy that is generated and play with your bodies—this is why it's called foreplay. If strong emotions arise, allow time for them to be processed. Intimacy and enjoyment rather than intercourse and orgasm are the goals of true lovemaking. Progress at a pace that is completely safe for you, communicating any fear or discomfort to your partner. Trust your intuition and the signals from your body as to what is nourishing to you, and do not cross boundaries because of some preconceived expectation. If your relationship is close enough to have physical intimacy, it is close enough for you to feel free to communicate your emotional needs.

If the cancer or its treatment has resulted in structural changes to your sexual organs, discuss your concerns with your physician so you can have accurate information about any physical limitations that you should be aware of. Most doctors have not received extensive training in discussing issues of sexuality but are able to competently address questions when the subject is raised. Since your doctor will probably not initiate the conversation, it becomes your responsibility to ask the questions that are of concern to you.

Acknowledge your vulnerability, which is the essence of true intimacy. As in every other aspect of life, cancer offers the opportunity to heal at deeper levels of our minds and our bodies. Sexuality is inextricably woven into the fabric of life and can be a profound source of healing energy when approached with reverence.

Colon Cancer—The Silent Obstructor

I am the son of the first fish who climbed ashore,
but the news has not yet reached my bowels.

W. S. MERWIN

At age sixty-four, Jonathan Hilms III was a good old boy. He believed that real men ate meat, used his double Scotch to relax at night, and shunned anything that was inconsistent with his model of a classic, hard-driving American businessman. When he saw his physician for heartburn that was awakening him at night, he expected a quick prescription for some antacid medication, but agreed to a more thorough examination at his doctor's urging. When his stool showed trace amounts of blood, he was convinced it was his ulcer acting up. Reluctantly, he complied with his doctor's recommendation to look at his entire digestive tract for the source of blood. During a colonoscopy, a small malignant polyp was discovered in his large bowel, which was easily and completely removed. Despite this scare, Mr. Hilms resumed his long-standing lifestyle, now even more confident that American know-how could accomplish anything.

We take justifiable pride in the ability of our medical system to make early diagnoses. Mammography, PSA levels, and tests that detect microscopic quantities of blood in our stools enable us catch cancers at earlier stages than ever before. These advances in early detection have given us a false sense of security that, simply stated, runs something like this: I don't really need to make changes in my lifestyle because modern medicine will patch me back together if I become ill. Fortunately, with regard to colon cancer, many cases detected early enough are curable, but I am certain that few people facing this illness would trade a cure for prevention.

Lately I've been thinking about the age-old adage "An ounce of prevention is worth a pound of cure," and realize that there is another level to this saying. Of course, it is better and less expensive to prevent a fire from igniting in your house than trying to put it out once it has started. The other side to this maxim is the recognition that tools that can be effective in prevention may be less potent once the problem has arisen. For example, with colon cancer, it is clear that diet plays an important role in raising our risk. It is less certain how powerful an impact nutritional approaches can have once the cancer has established itself. Holistic approaches offer tremendous value in improving the quality of life in people with cancer. My hope is that if you are fortunate to reach the point where your bout with cancer is behind you, you will continue to embrace these health-enhancing and life-supporting behaviors for the benefits they bring on a daily basis, whether or not you are facing a serious illness. Begin them now for the value they bring in helping you cope with the challenges of cancer. Continue them for the rest of your life for the value they bring in helping you to realize and experience the mystery and grandeur of living life as a human being.

The Challenge of Colon Cancer

Among the most common malignancies in the Western world, colon cancer is relatively rare in India, Latin America, and Africa. The rate of colon cancer in Connecticut is almost ten times greater than the incidence in Bombay, India. The highest rates in the world are found in North America, Australia, and New Zealand. Interestingly, for reasons that are not clear, the lowest age-adjusted incidence in the world is found in non-Jewish Israelis; their risk of colon cancer is between one-third and one-fourth that of native-born Israeli Jews.[15]

As we've seen with other tumors, regardless of the incidence in one's home country, the risk for colon cancer approaches the rate of the destination country the longer one resides there. If you were born in Japan, China, or Latin America and migrate to the United States, by the time you have been living here for twenty years, your risk is very close to that of a native-born American, regardless of your ethnic origin. In general, people living in industrialized countries have higher rates of colon cancer than those living in developing countries, and city dwellers are at higher risk than people living in rural areas. Once again, the primary culprit seems to be our affluent eating habits. Studies have consistently shown that a low-fiber, high-animal-fat diet directly contributes to the development of colon cancer. In societies where vegetables are the mainstay of meals and red meat is rare, colon cancer is proportionately rare.

We don't usually think about our bowels. As long as they are not calling for any attention, they are far away both anatomically and psychologically from our daily concerns. The very word "bowels" conjures up images of deep, dark, dank, and shadowy realms. And yet, almost everything we eat is eventually processed in our colon, which is constantly exposed to the by-products of our consumption. Considering that the contents of our bowels are all that remain after we have absorbed all that is nourishing, it should not be surprising that exposure to these toxins over years of life can eventually cause sickness. The undigested products of nutrition that enter into the fecal stream carry a host of carcinogens. Cholesterol, bile acids, and altered animal proteins have all been shown to have the capability of creating mutations in our colonic DNA. Frying, grilling, and smoking meats seem to have a particular penchant for activating carcinogens.

Countering the Threats

How do we mitigate the effect of these waste chemicals on our poor vulnerable gut cells? Reduce your intake of animal fat and increase the fruits, vegetables, and whole grains in your diet. The abundant fiber in this nutritional program acts through several possible mechanisms. High fiber speeds up the movement of food through our digestive tracts so that carcinogens have less time to do their evil work. Fiber also seems to bind potential cancer-causing chemicals, rendering them less dangerous. Finally, fiber can alter the populations of bacteria in our guts which contribute to the creation of certain carcinogens.

In addition to fiber, the antioxidant vitamins C and E and beta-carotene have been explored as possible guardians of the colon. All have been suggested to provide some protection, but the results have not been universally positive. In laboratory studies, vitamin A has been shown to accelerate the death of colon cancer cells in animals, although we do not know whether this happens in people.[16] Our trace element friend selenium (see chapter 4) has also been shown to have a protective effect in animal models of colon cancer.[17]

Other choices that create an environment unfavorable to colon cancer include avoiding cigarettes and spending less time as a couch potato and more time exercising. People who are physically active have about half the risk of colon cancer of people who rarely perform physical activity. One of the explanations for this dramatic benefit is that exercise stimulates the release of natural chemicals that speed up movement through the digestive tract, reducing the time that potential carcinogens have to harm the lining cells of the colon. If your job does not require you to be physically active on a regular basis, start moving your body today.

The Benefits of Dairy

Whenever I speak about the role of dairy products as part of a balanced diet, I usually encounter people who have very strong feelings on this subject. In certain nutritional circles, dairy is right next to cyanide in its potential toxicity in human beings. And yet, according to Ayurveda, dairy products are considered among the most health-promoting foods available to us. Studies looking at the role of dairy products on colon cancer have consistently suggested that they confer a protective effect. The main benefits of dairy products seem to be through the calcium and vitamin D they provide to our bodies.[18] Calcium is thought to bind with potentially carcinogenic bile acids and fatty acids, turning them into harmless soaps that will not irritate our intestinal linings. Vitamin D, which plays an important part in calcium metabolism, appears to have its own role in regulating the ways that cells divide. In areas that receive more daily sunlight, people have higher concentrations of vitamin D and lower rates of colon cancer. Thus milk products provide double value when it comes to colon cancer.

I understand the concerns that environmentally sensitive people have about dairy products. We do not, in general, treat our cows with exemplary displays of compassion and care. However, a growing number of dairies are committed to improving the treatment of dairy cows, allowing them to have regular access to open grazing lands and avoiding the use of hormones. Although organic milk from these dairies comes with a premium price, I encourage you to spend the extra money to support these farmers. It makes sense to me that the ethical treatment of animals can only enhance the health-promoting benefits of the products they provide to us.

Gut Feelings

Healthy digestion, absorption, and elimination are the keys to well being. If you are facing colon cancer, your elimination zone is demanding your attention. Although your tendency may be to divert your awareness away from the region of illness, bringing your attention to your bowels can have a powerful healing effect. I encourage you to try the following exercise:

~ Warm up a small bottle of castor oil by running it under hot tap water. Also, have a thin cotton towel and heating pad or hot water bottle available. Using the warm castor oil, gently massage your

belly in a clockwise direction. Making certain that your hands
are warm, begin at your right lower abdomen, moving up along
your right side to the area of your liver under your ribs. Then
massage across the upper part of your belly, from your right to
your left side, then down along the left side into your pelvis.
Begin with a light stroking motion, gradually pressing slightly
deeper with each cycle. If you have had recent surgery, caress
very gently around the incision, avoiding any fresh wound
sites. Close your eyes as you are massaging your belly and visualize golden, healing energy flowing into your abdomen.
Envision your digestive tract comfortably moving food along
its path, absorbing nutrients, and eliminating toxins. In the
warmth and light of your healing energy, visualize the melting
away of any obstacles to normal digestion, absorption, and
elimination.

~   Now, lay the thin towel over your abdomen and cover it with
the warm heating pad or water bottle. Make certain that the
temperature is not too hot. Allow the warmth to permeate your
belly, envisioning it as golden healing light. With each breath,
release the tension you have been carrying in your gut and replace it with relaxation, comfort, and trust. As you bring this exercise to a close, make a commitment to allow only healthy,
nourishing food into your body to facilitate the healing of your
digestive tract.

Integrating the Information

If you are facing colon cancer, what can you do for yourself to facilitate
the healing process? First and foremost, follow the advice of your health
care provider. Diagnosed and treated early, a cancerous colon tumor is
curable. To create as healthy a digestive environment as possible, reduce
your intake of animal fat and increase your consumption of fiber-rich
fresh fruits and vegetables. Reduce the amount of fried foods you are eating and be certain to get at least 1,500 milligrams of calcium in your diet
each day. During your treatments, it is prudent to take a good daily antioxidant vitamin formula with adequate vitamin C (1 gram), vitamin E
(300 IU) and beta-carotene (25,000 IU), but over the longer term, you
should be able to ensure adequate vitamin intake if you follow a vegetable,
fruit, and whole-grain-rich diet. Drink plenty of fresh fruit and vegetable

juices each day, along with warm ginger tea. Begin a daily exercise program, preferably outdoors where you can connect with your natural environment. Use the immediacy of this illness to look at all the issues in your life—relationships, job, spirituality—and give yourself permission to make choices that will bring you greater love, happiness, and fulfillment.

Conscious Healing

The path to wholeness requires perseverance, flexibility, and openness. As you travel along your healing journey, you'll have new experiences and uncover fresh information that will deepen your wisdom of life. The challenge in this process, as in all of life, is to extract that which is beneficial and release that which is not. To assess the many recommendations that will cross your path, you will need to use both your heart and your head. The greatest part of this book has been devoted to sharing the approaches that I have found useful in accessing and interpreting the wisdom we carry within. What our hearts and guts feel about something can help guide us to healthier choices. Our body's intelligence is profound and powerful.

We also have the power of discrimination, which enables us to critically analyze and assess information that may be useful for our health. We are living in an information age and through technology have instantaneous access to the thinking of more people around the world than ever before in the history of humankind. I encourage you to take full advantage of this network of energy and information and continue to expand your knowledge about your illness and the healing approaches available. There are a number of valuable sources of reliable health information accessible through the World Wide Web.[19] One of the most useful sites is the National Library of Medicine, which can be found at *www.nlm.nih.gov* on the Internet. You can enter the PubMed section and request a search for the topic you are interested in, such as "prostate cancer and diet" or "breast cancer and beta-carotene." Another powerful and highly reliable source of cancer information is available through a site collaboratively produced by the International Cancer Information Center (ICIC), the National Cancer Institute (NCI), and the Office of Cancer Communications, known as CancerNet, which can be found at *http://cancernet.nci.nih.gov* on the Web. If you do not have a computer, you can receive help from the National Cancer Institute Cancer Information Service, at (800) 4–CANCER [(800) 422–6237].

Keep your mind and your body open to receiving guidance from all helpful sources and avoid creating arbitrary boundaries between holistic and allopathic approaches. As localized networks of conscious energy within the vast ocean of energy and information, we have an intrinsic right to the storehouse of healing wisdom from around the world and across the ages. In the realm of mind-body medicine we can access healing information using our minds and our bodies for the benefit of both.

Commitment to Wholeness

Our bodies are the end products of our experiences and interpretations. To change our bodies, we need to change our experiences. Make a commitment to change your life in the direction of greater love and caring for yourself and those close to you.

1. I commit to becoming an expert on the type of cancer I am facing so I can be confident that all potentially successful treatment options have been considered.

2. I commit to establishing a healthy line of communication with my health care providers, based upon mutual trust, respect, and partnership.

3. I will at all times treat my body with love, compassion, and reverence, appreciating its remarkable resiliency in the face of adversity.

CHAPTER 15

The Unknown Destination

Facing Our Fear of Death by Embracing Life

Until we have made peace with death, we cannot make peace with life. Until we have accepted the whole reality of life, we cannot live with meaningful satisfaction and mature purpose.—RABBI ALVIN I. FINE

While you do not know life, how can you know about death?—CONFUCIUS

Facing cancer means facing your mortality. Your doctor may reassure you that the tumor is contained and that your chances of a complete remission are excellent. You may be informed that the cancer has spread but your treatment has a good chance of being successful. Sadly, you may be told that modern medical therapy has little to offer and that your time is limited. Whatever the direct communication you are hearing, you are also receiving messages that each of us hears but represses on a daily basis: life is delicate . . . life is brief . . . cherish your time here . . . celebrate life.

Cancer brings into focus the fundamental questions of life: Why am I here? What is the meaning of my life? Is there a God? Does he or she really care about me? What happens when I die? Will I still exist in some form after I have left my body? Is there heaven and hell? Is there reincarnation? Most of us have asked these questions at some time during our lives, and the answers are different for each of us. Our lives are a journey of discovery in which we pick up fragments of truth that we fit into our picture of life, like pieces in a jigsaw puzzle. At some point along the way we get a sense of the big picture and, from that time on, are forever transformed.

We are on this miraculous spaceship together, traveling through the universe. We board this vehicle at the time of birth, exit it at the time of death, and along the way we rejoice and suffer, win and lose, learn and forget. When facing a serious illness, urgency approaches, and yet the urgency has actually been there all along. We only need to watch the evening news to realize that we can never really predict when our time is up. A person facing cancer may outlive someone with no apparent illness who succumbs in an automobile accident. However, the inevitability of our limited time on this plane is brought to the forefront when we are forced to face cancer.

Responses to Death

It is natural to feel fear when facing loss. The life impulse is hardwired into our being, and whether we are a one-celled amoeba or a complex hominid, we are designed for self-preservation. It is a rare human soul who is so enlightened that he or she faces death with total equanimity. Most of us go through a process of release in which we surrender those aspects of ourselves that are ephemeral, while we become increasingly clear about our essential natures. The compassionate healer and researcher Elizabeth Kübler-Ross described five psychological stages that people go through when facing a life-threatening illness: denial, anger, bargaining, depression, and acceptance.[1] Although it has never been convincingly demonstrated that this sequence is accurate or universal, her description of the dying process focused attention on a topic that had been sorely neglected in our society. I have found it most beneficial to use Dr. Kübler-Ross's five stages as a framework for exploring the many different feelings that people experience when they are confronting cancer. There is a vast array of responses to facing our mortality. Every response is valid and important for the people experiencing them and must be acknowledged in order for them to feel complete. Let's explore an expanded repertoire of responses to facing our death and see what lessons each has to offer.

Disbelief

When something unexpectedly bad happens to us, it is natural at first to doubt the reality of it. This is true whether we are talking about being fired from a job, finding that our wallet was stolen, or learning discouraging news about our health. The shock of the threatening information numbs us emotionally in a similar way that physical trauma often triggers a state of anesthesia. This is a protective response that gives us time to digest the message at a pace we can handle. Some amount of denial is to be anticipated whenever we receive overwhelming, unanticipated information—either good or bad. If you receive a phone call informing you that you won a major cash prize, you might respond, "I don't believe it!" In the original scheme proposed by Dr. Kübler-Ross, she described denial as a common first stage. It is fairly rare that I see people maintaining a state of denial, except when the information is so insensitively presented that the person literally shuts down, becoming incapable of directly addressing the pressing issues facing them.

> After three months of a hacking cough, Mrs. Rose sought attention from her doctor, who ordered a chest X ray due to her prior smoking history. The next day she received a message on her answering machine telling her to make an appointment with a lung specialist as soon as possible. She immediately panicked and called her doctor, who told her there was a concerning "spot" on her lung that needed further investigation. She was unable to see the specialist for several days, by which time she was terrified. When he entered the examination room, his first words were, "You understand that you'll need an operation to remove the lung cancer, followed by radiation and chemotherapy to reduce your chances of metastasis." She was so shocked she doesn't remember anything else that was told to her that day. When she came to the Chopra Center, she was adamant that she would not undergo any medical treatment and wanted only "natural alternative" approaches. Fortunately, after we won her trust over several days, she was willing to see our pulmonary consultant, who presented her with the therapeutic options that would maximize her chances for the best outcome while supporting her use of complementary mind-body approaches.

Disbelief and denial are healthy initial components of coping with cancer and the potential for dying that it brings. As with every aspect of human nature, there is an appropriate time and place for denial and a time to go beyond it. Seek out health care providers and supporters who can help you process the painful bits of information that you are facing at a pace that is appropriate for you. On the other hand, don't allow denial to interfere with making the choices that will take you to your highest level of integration.

Hope

Hope is an essential aspect of life and can take many forms. Most people facing cancer hope they will be cured of their disease. If not cured, they hope for a prolonged life. If not a prolonged life, they hope for a life that is meaningful and of high quality. At some point, hope shifts from staying alive at all costs to hoping for a peaceful death. A good doctor will always present information in a way that is honest and supports the possibility of hope. If every time you leave your doctor you feel disheartened, communicate your feelings honestly, and if necessary, search for another caregiver.

Hope is the window that keeps our hearts open to the gifts of life. Each day that you awaken, express your hopes for that day silently or aloud. They do not have to be profound. You may hope for something as simple as a visit from your friend, the opportunity to feel the sun on your face for another day, the pleasure of hearing the robins sing, relief from pain for several hours, or simply having a good bowel movement. Once you have expressed your hopes, set your intentions in motion by mobilizing your support team to help you realize your desires. Pray to your God for those things that are likely as well as for the miraculous.

Anger

Although anger has been considered a standard stage of coming to terms with life-threatening illness, I have found it more common for people with cancer to have difficulty accepting, experiencing, and expressing their anger. Anger is a natural reaction to being hurt and there is no question that cancer hurts our bodies and our minds. Directed anger can be empowering and invaluable in triggering profound emotional release. Undirected anger can be destructive and can compound the anguish that you and your loved ones are experiencing.

Take time to get in touch with your anger. With whom are you angry? A friend or family member who has not provided the support you have been needing? Your doctor or health care provider, for not taking enough time with you or not having adequate tools to heal you? God, for creating a world that includes sickness and death? You, for your perceived sins of omission or commission? Write about your anger without filtering or judging yourself. Then perform some action to help express and release it. Throw stones at the ocean, take a plastic bat and pound a pillow, dance in a screaming frenzy. Once the emotional charge has dissipated, express yourself in spoken words or writing, taking responsibility for your feelings of anger. If you give yourself permission to feel and release your rage in a manner that does not hurt others or yourself, a tremendous amount of energy and life force will become available to you.

Frustration

Frustration is an almost universal experience, for it is the result of our imperfect and often inadequate tools available to treat cancer. Most people with cancer feel the "big" frustration that the disease refuses to disappear from their pure will of wanting it to be gone. However, it is often the little frustrations that can trap us in whirlpools of unnecessary distress. Your clothes don't fit as well, your hair isn't growing back fast enough, the insurance company is being difficult, you have to wait too long at your doctor's appointments—these are the day-to-day hassles that can erode your semblance of equanimity. These annoyances are also opportunities for practicing consciousness-based living. Patience is considered a virtue, because it is not something that comes easily or naturally to many of us. As a naturally impatient person, I have found this "Patience Meditation" to be helpful in maintaining my center when I have little control over my environment.

~ When you notice you are feeling frustrated while waiting for something that you know will eventually come, use your internal sensations to enter into present-moment awareness. Become aware of your impatience, and bring your attention into your body. Notice where you are experiencing tension and consciously breathe into the area. With each breath, release the tension you are holding, noticing any pressure in your neck, jaw, shoulders, back, or legs. Pay particular attention to the resistance in your chest, purposely releasing and freeing your breathing with slow deep inhalations and exhalations. Shift your internal dialogue from one of anxious anticipation to one of appreciation for the moment of quietness you are being afforded.

If you practice this process, you may notice that situations you previously associated with frustration are now considered small gifts. Waiting for something that we know will come provides a brief respite from our constant need to decide what our next step is. If you are waiting in your doctor's office, you can enjoy the pause between actions by practicing patience meditation. The time will pass much more quickly, and you will have transformed an uncomfortable experience into a gratifying one.

Regret

Regret is one of the most painful emotions we can experience. Looking back at our lives, all of us can recall times and circumstances when we wished we could play back the video and try a second take. We may wish we had taken a different path, made a different choice, used different words to communicate something, taken more risk, or spent more time with those we loved. Do not chastise yourself with regrets, for at any time in the past, you were doing your best, given the level of consciousness available to you at the time. You have an opportunity right now to make a difference in the quality of your life by healing with someone with whom you have shared pain. There is a beautiful expression in the Jewish Day of Atonement service that says, "For transgressions against God, the Day of Atonement atones, but for transgressions of one human being against another, the Day of Atonement does not atone until they have made peace with one another."[2]

Facing death is your greatest opportunity to make peace with your life, for you really have nothing to lose and everything to gain. Seize the opportunity of your dying to forgive those who have wronged you through their words or actions, intentionally or unintentionally, and ask for the forgiveness of those whom you may have harmed.

Negotiation

Originally described as bargaining by Dr. Kübler-Ross, negotiation is the process whereby a dying person seeks to make a better deal with fate. This is a very basic psychological process that most of us have used during our lives. "Please, God, if you help me make the cheerleading squad, I promise I'll never torture my little brother again." When facing a serious illness, the negotiation may sound like "If I can just live until my son graduates from college or my new grandchild is born, I will stop pressuring my daughter to get married." And indeed, several studies have shown that we are capable of prolonging our lives while waiting for a meaningful life event. The mortality among Jews dips sharply the week before Passover, rising a proportionate amount the week after the holiday.[3] Similarly, the mortality among Chinese people falls substantially in the week before the Harvest Moon Festival, peaking the following week.[4]

These findings are true only for groups that invest important significance in the event. The meanings we attribute to life events directly impact our healing systems.

Negotiation can be an important component in healing body, mind, and soul. It adds substantial leverage to a life change if you believe you are bargaining with fate. People with cancer are often willing to try new ways to think, speak, and act that they would have casually dismissed when healthy. Most are willing to do whatever is possible to stay alive, including experimental treatment protocols, mind-body interventions, alternative therapies, emotional clearing, and spiritual practices, if they think it may help. Major lifestyle changes are the bargaining chips that modern cancer patients are willing to offer in the hope that time can be gained. I see this response as an opportunity for personal transformation, for it again allows you to make a conscious choice as to how you wish to live your life. Although your motivation may be for the sake of living longer, bringing awareness into every moment provides tangible benefits now. Living fully is our ultimate birthright, even though it may take facing our death to openly embrace this truth.

Grief

If despite your best efforts, you find you are losing your struggle with cancer, it is natural to feel grief. Sadness in the face of loss is intrinsic to human experience, and there is no greater loss than our individuality. Loss of time, loss of control, loss of comfort, loss of independence—these are real losses that we face as we approach our end of life, and it is normal to feel sorrow. There is no easy detour around this anguish, and although it doesn't feel good to be with your pain, it is essential that you allow yourself the time and space to experience it. I recommend you give yourself the opportunity to cry openly and freely every day. It is sad that we cannot stay on earth until we have accomplished everything we would like. It is sad that we are here for such a short time. It is sad that we may not see our children or grandchildren grow up, but is not our fault that dying is an inevitable feature of life. Death is the eternal stalker, driving us to live fully.

If you know you are dying from your illness, embrace your sadness and share your sadness with your friends and loved ones. Tell them how you would like to deal with your dying process. Many people are uncertain or uncomfortable about how to act around someone who is dying, and although it is not your job to make them comfortable, it is useful to give them permission to express their sadness, fears, and concerns. It is okay to think about dying and it's okay to talk about dying. Thinking and talking about death will not hasten its arrival. It will deepen your connection to those with whom you are going through the process.

Dying is not a sign of failure, as it is the quality, not the quantity, of our lives that matters. Great saints die, nasty evildoers die, and all of us in between die. Pure vegetarians die, hard-core meat eaters die, and all of us in between die. Devoutly religious people die, devout atheists die, and all of us in between die. In your sadness you are grieving not only for yourself but for every person who has ever lived. But the deepest sadness is felt for those who fail to fully cherish the miraculous opportunity to be a human being.

The good news is that it is never too late to embrace the moment. Share your heart and spirit with those around you, and your life has meaning. We cannot change the events of the past, we can only change our interpretation of them. If we have learned from our past, our lives have been of value to ourselves and to all humanity.

Surrender

There will come a time in each of our lives when we no longer wish to fight. A noble surrender is most likely when we know in our heart of hearts that we have given our best effort. An incalculable number of prior events have contributed to your life at this moment and to struggle against the river of life is to struggle against all of nature. There is a time to swim and a time to allow the current to carry us to the next phase. In our surrender, we are only acknowledging what has been true all along— that nature exercises the ultimate and supreme power in our lives. Surrender is not the same as resignation, for there is a reluctance in resignation that is not present in true surrender. Acceptance follows surrender, dawning as we relinquish our attachments and allow the unifying force of spirit to flow through us. Surrender is the recognition that letting go will bring us what we have been searching for our entire lives—peace.

In the process of releasing, we accelerate the disengagement between what is transitory and what is real. That which is real persists and is independent of time and circumstance. That which is ephemeral has a beginning, middle, and end. Our bodies, emotions, relationships, beliefs, and possessions have cycles of birth, maintenance, and dissolution. Therefore, if we have sought to establish security and comfort in our life solely through our possessions and positions, we will naturally feel insecure and uncomfortable as we find these objects of identification separating from us. Although the great sages of the world have consistently told us we are in this world but not of this world, most of us still have attachments, and it hurts as these bonds are separated. And yet, even as you are experiencing the pain and the loss, you can see that the experiencer—the one who is having the experience—remains. This witnessing presence upholds the continuity to your life. It is the essence of who you are.

According to Ayurveda, human beings are composed of layers of consciousness. Our most dense layer is our physical body, comprised of matter and energy. Subtler than our physical sheath is our emotional layer, embodying our feelings about ourselves and the world. Still subtler is our belief layer, in which we carry our opinions, or those ideas that we hold to be true. Even closer to our core are the seeds of memory and desire that have been driving our lives. Each of us enters this world with our own unique blueprint for what we need to bring pleasure, satisfaction, and fulfillment into our lives. Finally, at the heart of our existence is that which underlies, supports, and actually becomes all the other layers of our being. This is our true nature, our ground state of existence, our spirit. This is who we really are, because this is that aspect that has never been born and therefore can never die. The Upanishads beautifully express this essential truth:

> The all-knowing Self was never born.
> Nor will it die. Beyond cause and effects,
> This Self is eternal and immutable.
> When the body dies, the Self does not die.
> If the slayer believes that he can slay
> Or the slain believes that he can be slain,
> Neither knows the truth. The eternal Self
> Slays not, nor is ever slain.[5]

As we advance through the dying process, we shed our attachments to our nonessential layers. A beautiful woman or a handsome man lose their attachment to physical appearance, no longer identifying themselves with their hair, face, or figure. Then they relinquish their identification with their activity in the world. A president of a corporation resigns from his position of authority; an attorney loses her attachment to her role as a litigator. As our withdrawal from individuality progresses, we release our strong emotions as judgment, blame, and resentment dissolve. Anger toward an ex-spouse, parent, or sibling is transformed into acceptance, forgiveness, and love. Relinquishing attachment to our layer of belief, our opinions lose their hold as we accept and embrace the ambiguity of life. Our perspective broadens as we realize that this plane is characterized by the coexistence of opposites. As we surrender all those aspects by which we defined our lives, we come to understand that these attachments were simply constructs of our ego. In the dissolution of individuality, universality dawns.

Gratitude

Although the thought of dying suddenly from cardiac arrest during sleep has a certain appeal, the lack of time to prepare and make peace with friends and loved ones is the downside of a quick exit. As more people choose to live and die consciously, I am seeing people who reach a very blissful state even while their bodies are experiencing progressive entropy. A state of acceptance, peace, and gratitude infuses their being, so that even though they may be experiencing some physical pain, they are not suffering. Along with this state of peace and gratitude, there is wisdom. The wisdom is usually expressed as a profound insight into the unity of life.

> Mr. Alexander had been through a difficult year with his colon cancer. After his initial surgery showed that the tumor had extended into the surrounding tissues, he underwent a protracted course of chemotherapy. Just as he was adjusting to the need for a colostomy, it was discovered that he had metastases in his liver. After a brief course of experimental chemotherapy, he decided he had had enough medicine and spent several weeks at an alternative cancer clinic in Mexico. When it became obvious to him that his cancer was progressing, he visited us at the Chopra Center. He was not looking for a cure; rather, he was hoping for some help in preparing for his death.
>
> During his week with us, Mr. Alexander learned meditation, reporting that while experiencing an expanded state of awareness he was pain-free for the first time in months. He found the sacred space guided meditation to be particularly meaningful, believing the celestial being he visualized to be his guardian angel. Realizing that he had some healing to do with his children, he made a commitment to clear with them when he arrived back home. For the first time in his life, he gave himself permission to simply be, without pressure to be goal-oriented. He created his own repertoire of music and aromas that he associated with his peaceful state of acceptance.

I spoke to Mr. Alexander a month later, by which time he had become essentially bedridden. Despite his obvious physical discomfort, he told me that he had never felt so safe and trusting in the universe. Although he had previously been a man uncomfortable expressing his feelings, he said that he now realized how much he loved his family and his life, and was very grateful for the time he had been given. He had never considered himself a particularly religious person, but now understood that God created the world as an expression of love and that ultimately love was the only real truth in life.

Two days later his wife called to tell me he had passed on in his sleep. She told me that he seemed to be truly happy during his final days, and to her surprise, despite the anguish of watching him fade, whenever she sat with him and held his hand, she also felt safe and happy.

Each person's dying process is as unique as each person's life. The experiences described above are neither universal or complete. People will often go back and forth between experiences of surrender and acceptance and feelings of anguish and grief. It is not easy to shed our mortal coil, and there is no one right way to die. Open your heart to the love around you, and allow it to carry you to a place of peace.

Rituals of Release

I recently attended the funeral of a close family member. After the standard prayers were said at the graveside service, several people who had been close to this man spoke about the value he had added to their lives. Beautiful stories were told of his determination and vitality in the face of a protracted illness. A common theme was how his love of music and the arts had inspired many people. After the service, another relative and I discussed how we often fail to tell people how we really feel about them until after they are gone. We can take advantage of the dying process to speak openly from our hearts, so that we do not have regrets at the time of death.

If you feel prepared to do so, envision how you would like your final days to be. Where do you want to die? Who do you want to be with you? Ask your friends and loved ones to create the space for your passing. It is an honor to lovingly assist someone in dying and an opportunity for deepening spirituality. Don't deprive those who care of the opportunity to be there for you in your final days.

Rituals after our passing are for the sake of our survivors. In every human culture around the world since time immemorial, a funeral ceremony serves two purposes—it honors the deceased and provides support for those grieving. Imagine what you would like people to hear from you when you are gone. It may be reciting your favorite poem, playing your favorite music, or reading a beautiful prayer. These rituals help survivors maintain their connection with the spirit of their beloved. They help to create meaning in the lives of the people you have loved. I see them as the emotional equivalent of a will. Your final message to your loved ones is part of the legacy of your heart.

The Next Step

What happens after we exhale our last breath? This question has been explored within the province of religious and spiritual traditions but, until fairly recently, was resolutely avoided by most scientists. Then in 1975, Dr. Raymond Moody published his book *Life After Life*, describing the near-death experiences of 150 patients.[6] These were people who had temporary cessation of vital functions, usually due to a major trauma, suicide attempt, or cardiac arrest. Although not every person reported the full range of experiences, Moody found a remarkable degree of similarity in people's accounts. Following his report, a number of other physicians and psychologists were inspired to question people who had been resuscitated and described nearly identical findings.[7, 8]

I find these reports fascinating, inspiring, and extremely familiar. A near-death experience has several distinctive features. In the earliest stage, people report a deep sense of peace and calm. They often comment that words are inadequate to describe the intensity of their feelings of comfort. Statements such as "I had a feeling of total peace . . . I wasn't frightened any more," or "All I felt was warmth and the most extreme comfort I have experienced," are common.[9, 10]

The second stage of many near-death experiences involves separation from the body. Often termed an out-of-body experience, people commonly describe viewing their body and the people around it from a distance. A man whose heart stopped during an operation reported upon his recovery, "I remember being up in the air looking down . . . and seeing myself on the operating table with all the people around working on me.

What sticks in my mind mostly, were the colors. Everything in that operating room was a very brilliant, bright color."[9]

The next stage for many people involves traveling through a dark space, often described as a tunnel. Although as children we usually associate darkness with fear, most people with near-death experiences describe the darkness as comforting and safe. A young woman whose heart stopped later described her experience: "I became less and less able to see and feel. Presently, I was going down a long black tunnel with a tremendous alive sort of light bursting in at the end. I shot out of the tunnel into this light."[11]

Experiencing the light after moving through the darkness is a component of near-death experiences around the world. The light is usually identified with a celestial presence, which varies, depending upon one's cultural or religious background. A Christian will often identify the light with Christ, a person of the Jewish faith may experience it as an angel, and a Hindu might see the light as a familiar deity. Approaching the light, people often report the experience of seeing their lives in review, not from the perspective of judgment as much as an opportunity for learning. Encounters with loved ones who have previously died are sometimes reported during this phase, where they usually serve to guide the person through the experience. This is also the time that some decision about whether to go back is made. Although at the beginning of the process, many people are reluctant about leaving their lives, by this stage, the beauty and rapture of the light is so intense that people feel disappointed when they find themselves coming back into their bodies. An open-heart surgery patient described her experience of the light: "It was like all of a sudden I could feel this whole feeling of love and joy. It was all around me. My eyes were automatically drawn to the side and I saw this circle of light off in the distance. I'll never forget it. And I could feel this love just coming from that light. It was all around me."[12]

The last phase of the near-death experience is entering into the light, in which people relate inexpressible beauty. The colors, sensations, and sounds are described as celestial or heavenly. A gentleman I cared for who had a near-death encounter from a drug overdose reported his experience of merging into the light:

> I was transported to a plane of unearthly beauty. All of my pain evaporated and I felt the inherent perfection of creation. I was infused with a divine light that seemed to be concentrated love of an intensity I had never before experienced or imagined. I saw

within this light, the entire universe being created and dissolved like a fountainhead spewing forth the world out of pure being. I felt that I merged with the Creator and understood that despite my struggles, everything was as it was supposed to be. The light was so pure and clear, I had the thought, "This is why it is called enlightenment." I didn't want to leave, and though I was told later that I had been "gone" for less than two minutes, I felt I had been beyond time.

Not everyone who has a near-death encounter reports any or all of these experiences, but they are far from rare. In most studies, about half of people who are questioned after resuscitation report some of the above elements. A fascinating recent report in the English journal *The Lancet* found that the closer a person was to actually dying, the more likely they were to report experiencing the later stages of seeing or entering into the light.[13] It would seem to follow that if dying is a journey, fewer people would have gone to the farther realms and still returned to tell us about it. In a study of over one hundred people with near-death experiences by Dr. Kenneth Ring, only 10 percent reported entering into the light compared to 60 percent who felt the first stage of peace and well being.

What are we to make of these near-death experiences? Psychologists may suggest that these experiences are wishful imaginations born of ego defense mechanisms mobilized to protect our minds from the terror of annihilation. Neurophysiologists may suggest that these near-death experiences result from biochemical changes as a result of oxygen deprivation. Of course, none of us will really know what happens to us when we pass on until it is our turn. Personally, I am profoundly inspired and reassured by these images. The descriptions seem very familiar to me, as if I am carrying similar memories deep in my storehouse of impressions. The fact that many of the elements of the near-death experiences related by Westerners are also described by Australian aborigines, Native Americans, New Zealand Maoris, as well as people from China, India, and Guam supports its universality among human beings.[14]

It may be the Tibetan Buddhists who have chronicled the dying journey in greater detail than any other spiritual tradition. According to the *Tibetan Book of the Dead*, written by eighth-century Tibetan monks, we progress through six different stages over fifty days until we choose our next incarnation.[15] Exiting our bodies through the tops of our heads, we first experience the Primordial Clear Light in the transition phase known as Chi-ka'i Bardo. After a few days of adjusting to our nonphysical state, we pass through many different celestial realms until we eventually sink back into the physical plane. Those of us conscious enough to remain fully aware of our unbounded spiritual nature despite encountering the worlds of peaceful and wrathful deities reach perfect Buddhahood, liberated from the cycle of death and rebirth.

Buddhist students are encouraged to practice leaving the body in advanced meditation techniques known as Pho-ba. According to Tibetan Buddhism, the better prepared one is for the transition out of the body, the easier and less distressing is the process when the actual time of death arrives. Although the full Pho-ba practice requires guidance from an experienced teacher, try this simple guided meditation. Record your own voice softly while slowly reading the visualization, or ask a friend or family member to guide you through.

- ~ Become aware of your breathing, allowing your fear, pain, and resistance to release with each breath. With each exhalation, relax the muscles in your neck, shoulders, chest, abdomen, and back, allowing soothing, comfortable relaxation to fill your body. As you go deeper in your quietness, notice how your body becomes heavier. Let the weight of your body go as your awareness carries you to an event that occurred yesterday. Remember in detail the sounds, sights, and sensations of a situation in which you participated. Now recall some event that took place within the last year. Envision the sounds, sights, and sensations as you witness the circumstance.

- ~ Continue moving backward in time, stopping to review significant events in your life—a marriage, a divorce, the birth of child, the death of a loved one. For each situation, hear the sounds, feel the sensations, see the images. Now imagine back to the time when you were floating in your mother's womb. Envision the sounds, the sensations, and sights while you continue to move back to a time before you were conceived—free-floating spirit, looking at your parents and the environment into which you will be born. You are awareness that has not yet condensed into matter.

- ~ Now play your life forward, moving through your childhood, graduations, important relationships, jobs, and significant events until you are back to your present circumstance. Project forward into your future to the day that you will leave your body. Envision releasing your last breath. As you move out of your body, envision the scene of your final moments. Now envision a pure, clear light, growing brighter in your awareness. Feel the warmth, love, and bliss of this celestial energy enveloping your soul as you are transported to a divine realm. Hear the heavenly music, envision the beautiful celestial environment, feel the comfort and joy. You have arrived home to the source of your being.

~ Now, slowly, reorient to your current time and place, feeling the chair or bed you are on, hearing the sounds in the room, returning to your body.

You now know that your spirit is not localized in time or space. It has never been bound in the past and will never be bound in the future.

Returning to Wholeness

The hope of every person facing cancer is that as a result of modern chemotherapy, complementary techniques, alternative approaches, or a miracle, their illness is overcome and life returns to some degree of normality. Fortunately, many people realize this scenario. Modern medicine holds powerful weapons in the fight against illness, and mind-body approaches designed to amplify intrinsic healing energy help expand our therapeutic arsenal.

Yet, despite our best efforts and intentions, people with cancer die. If this is the ultimate outcome, I do not view it as failure. Our interpretation of our experiences creates our reality. Dying is a supreme opportunity for spiritual growth, for in the process of releasing our physical vessel, we learn that our true nature is holy. People frequently consider if they only had one year to live, how would they change their lives? Directly confronting our mortality impels us to live each day to its fullest, appreciating the simpler things that we usually take for granted when we believe we have all the time in the world.

As our separateness dissolves into unity, we recover our essential natures as nonmaterial beings composed of conscious energy. We are truly beings of light. In the ultimate stage of our healing, we move beyond fear, beyond pain, and beyond suffering. In our understanding and experience of our essential nature as spiritual beings created of love . . . we return to wholeness.

In front stretches the ocean of Peace.
O Helmsman, sail out to the open sea.
You will be my eternal companion—
Take, O take me in your arms.
The Pole-star will shine
Lighting the path to Eternity.
O Lord of Deliverance,
Your forgiveness, your mercy
Shall be my everlasting sustenance
On my journey to the shores of Eternity.
May the bonds of earth dissolve,
The mighty Universe take me to her arms,
And I come to know fearlessly
The Great Unknown.[16]

RABRINDRANATH TAGORE

Postscript

A recent paper in the *New England Journal of Medicine* lamented that despite billions of dollars spent over the last quarter century on cancer research, there has been no overall change in the age-adjusted mortality from this dreaded common disease.[1] This paper triggered a storm of energetic responses from cancer physicians and researchers, disputing the conclusion that we should spend more money on prevention, rather than focusing so much of our resources on treatment. Another recent report from the American Cancer Society suggested that largely as a result of prevention and early detection programs, we are seeing a slight reduction in the incidence and mortality of overall cancers in the United States.[2] I do not believe that the cause of reducing the suffering from cancer is well served by crossfire between prevention and treatment advocates within the cancer care community. I hope and believe that with the new scientific tools of molecular biology, genetic engineering, and immunotherapy we will see significant advances in our ability to diagnose and treat malignancies over the next quarter century. I also hope and believe that as a society we will recognize the role of lifestyle choices and environmental toxicity in the development of cancer and will collectively reduce our tolerance for impurity in our lives. It is my fervent desire that as a society we will increasingly accept and embrace the role of mind-body approaches in improving the quality of life of people facing serious illnesses.

I wrote this book with the intention of opening the door to a more expanded view of health and illness, life and death, that embraces body, mind, and spirit. Cancer cannot be effectively addressed if it is approached only from a materialistic perspective. A health problem that takes more lives in our society than any other illness besides heart disease is shouting a warning to us about how we are living. My hope is that as we collectively heed its message, cancer will not need to shout so loudly to get our attention.

I pray that those who are facing cancer and those who love those who are facing cancer find healing and peace in their lives. May the offerings contained in this book help relieve suffering while expanding love and wisdom.

Appendix

General Ayurvedic References

Chopra, D. 1991. *Perfect Health*. New York: Harmony Books.

Frawley, D. 1989. *Ayurvedic Healing—A Comprehensive Guide*. Salt Lake City, Utah: Passage Press.

Heyn, B. 1990. *Ayurveda—The Indian Art of Natural Medicine and Life Extension*. Rochester, Vt.: Healing Arts Press.

Joshi, S. V. 1997. *Ayurveda and Panchakarma*. Twin Lakes, Wis.: Lotus Press.

Lad, V. 1984. *Ayurveda—The Science of Self-Healing*. Santa Fe, N.Mex.: Lotus Press.

Ranade, S. 1993. *Natural Healing through Ayurveda*. Salt Lake City, Utah: Passage Press.

Rhyner, H. H. 1994. *Ayurveda—The Gentle Health System*. New York: Sterling Publishing.

Simon, D. 1997. *The Wisdom of Healing*. New York: Harmony Books.

Svoboda, R. E. 1992. *Ayurveda—Life, Health and Longevity*. London: Arkana Penguin Books.

Tiwari, M. 1995. *Ayurveda—Secrets of Healing*. Twin Lakes: Wis.: Lotus Press.

Notes

Introduction

1. Easwaren, E. 1987. *The Upanishads*. Petaluma, Calif.: Nilgiri Press, 1987, 191.

Chapter 1 ~ Understanding Cancer

1. Doll, R., and R. Peto. 1981. The causes of cancer: Quantitative estimates of avoidable risks of cancer in the United States today. *Journal of the National Cancer Institute* 66:1191–1308.
2. Carroll, K. K., and H. T. Kohr. 1975. Dietary fat in relation to tumorigenesis. *Progress in Biochemistry and Pharmacology* 10:308–353.
3. Phillips, R. L., L. Garfinkel, et al. 1980. Mortality among California Seventh-day Adventists for selected cancer sites. *Journal of the National Cancer Institute* 65:1097–1107.
4. Locke, F. B., and H. King. 1980. Cancer mortality risk among Japanese in the United States. *Journal of the National Cancer Institute* 65:1149–1156.
5. Berman, C. 1958. Primary carcinoma of the liver. *Advances in Cancer Research* 5:55–96.
6. Buell, P. 1973. Changing incidence of breast cancer in Japanese-American women. *Journal of the National Cancer Institute* 51:1479–1483.
7. Crisp, T. M., E. D. Clegg, and R. L. Cooper. 1997. Special report on environmental endocrine disruption: An effects assessment and analysis. Washington, D.C.: Risk Assessment Forum. U.S. Environmental Protection Agency, 1–116.

Chapter 2 ~ Eavesdropping on the Mind-Body Conversation

1. Salk, J. 1983. *Anatomy of Reality*. New York: Columbia University Press.
2. Cohen, S. 1991. Psychological stress and susceptibility to the common cold. *New England Journal of Medicine* 325:606–12.
3. Kiecolt-Glaser, J. K., R. Glaser, et al. 1986. Modulation of cellular immunity in medical students. *Journal of Behavioral Medicine* 9:5–21.
4. Linn, M. W., B. S. Linn, and J. Jensen. 1984. Stressful life events, dysphoric mood, and immune responsiveness. *Psychological Reports* 54:219–22.
5. Ader, R. 1975. Behaviorally conditioned immunosuppression. *Psychosomatic Medicine* 37:333–42.
6. Bovbjerg, D. H., and W. H. Redd. 1992. Anticipatory nausea and immune suppression in cancer patients receiving cycles of chemotherapy: Conditioned responses? In *Psychoneuroimmunology*, H. Schmoll, U. Tewews, and N. P. Plotnikoff, eds. Lewiston, N.Y.: Hoegrefe & Huber Publishers, 237–50.
7. Simonton, O. C., S. Matthews-Simonton, and J. Creighton. 1978. *Getting Well Again: A step-by-step self-help guide to overcoming cancer for patients and their families*. Los Angeles: J. P. Tarcher.
8. Spiegel, D., and S. Sands. 1983. Group therapy and hypnosis reduce metastatic breast carcinoma pain. *Psychosomatic Medicine* 45:333–39.
9. Spiegel, D., J. R. Bloom, et al. 1989. Effect of psychosocial treatment on survival of patients with metastatic breast cancer. *Lancet* 2:888–91.
10. Fawzy, F., N. Cousins, et al. 1990. A structured psychiatric intervention for cancer patients. *Archives of General Psychiatry* 47:720–25, 729–35.

Chapter 3 ~ Nutritional Healing

1. Armstrong, B., and R. Doll. 1975. Environmental factors and cancer incidence and mortality in different countries, with special reference to dietary practices. *International Journal of Cancer* 15:617–31.

2. Creasey, W. A. 1985. *Dietary fats: Diet and cancer.* Philadelphia: Lea & Febiger.

3. Kritchevsky, D., and D. M. Klurfeld. 1991. Dietary fiber and cancer. In *Cancer and Nutrition*, R. B. Alfin-Slater and D. Kritchevsky, eds. New York: Plenum Press, 211–220.

4. Bellman, S. 1983. Onion and garlic oils inhibit tumor promotion. *Carcinogenesis* 4:1063–65.

5. Alldrick, A. J. 1991. Diet and mutagenesis. In *Nutrition, Toxicity, and Cancer*, W. A. Creasey, ed. Boca Raton, Fla.: CRC Press, pp. 281–300.

6. Ji, B. T., W. H. Chow, et al. 1997. Green tea consumption and the risk of pancreatic and colorectal cancers. *International Journal of Cancer* 70:255–58.

7. Zheng, W., T. J. Doyle, et al. 1996. Tea consumption and cancer incidence in a prospective cohort study of postmenopausal women. *American Journal of Epidemiology* 144:175–82.

8. Clifford, A. J., S. E. Ebeler, et al. 1996. Delayed tumor onset in transgenic mice fed an amino acid-based diet supplemented with red wine solids. *American Journal of Clinical Nutrition* 64:748–56.

9. Carter, J. P., G. P. Saxe, et al. 1993. Hypothesis: Dietary management may improve survival from nutritionally linked cancers based on analysis of representative cases. *Journal of the American College of Nutrition* 12:209–26.

10. Gerson, M. 1977. *A Cancer Therapy: Result of fifty cases.* Del Mar, Calif.: Totality Books.

Chapter 4 ~ Heroic Biochemicals

1. Ames, B. N., M. K. Shigenaga, and T. M. Hagen. 1993. Oxidants, antioxidants, and degenerative diseases of aging. *Proceedings of the National Academy of Science (U.S.A.)* 90:7915–22.

2. Moertel, C. G., Flemming, T. R., et al. 1985. High dose vitamin C versus placebo in the treatment of patients with advanced cancer who have had no prior chemotherapy. *New England Journal of Medicine* 312:137–41.

3. Birt, D. F. 1986. Update on the effects of vitamins A, C, E and selenium on carcinogenesis. *Proceedings of the Society of Experimental Biology and Medicine* 183:311–20.

4. Jacob, R. A. 1994. Vitamin C. In *Modern Nutrition in Health and Disease*, 8th ed., M. E. Shils, J. A. Olson, and M. Shike, eds. Philadelphia: Lea & Febiger.

5. Shiilotri, P. G., and K. S. Bhat. 1977. Effect of megadoses of vitamin C on bactericidal activity of leukocytes. *American Journal of Clinical Nutrition* 30:1977–81.

6. Meydani, S. N., M. Meydani, et al. 1997. Vitamin E supplementation and in vivo immune response in healthy elderly subjects. *Journal of the American Medical Association* 277:1380–86.

7. Sanders, B. G., and K. Kline. 1995. Nutrition, immunology and cancer: An overview. In *Nutrition and Biotechnology in Heart Disease and Cancer*, J. B. Longenecker et al., eds. New York: Plenum Press.

8. Rock, C. L., R. A. Jacob, and P. E. Bowen. 1996. Update on the biological characteristics of the antioxidant micronutrients: Vitamin C, vitamin E, and the carotenoids. *Journal of the American Dietetic Association* 96:693–702.

9. Faure, H., C. Coudray, et al. 1996. 5-hydroxymethlyuracil excretion, plasma TBARS and plasma antioxidant vitamins in adriamycin-treated patients. *Free Radical Biology and Medicine* 20:979–83.

10. Chinery, R., J. A. Brockman, et al. 1997. Antioxidants enhance the cytotoxicity of chemotherapeutic agents in colorectal cancer. *Nature Medicine* 3:1233–41.

11. Bairati, I., F. Brochet, et al. 1996. Prevention of second primary cancer with vitamin supplementation in patients treated for head and neck cancers. *Bulletin du Cancer Radiotherapie* 83:12–16.

12. Tribble, D. L., and E. Frank. 1994. Dietary antioxidants, cancer, and atherosclerotic heart disease. *Western Journal of Medicine* 161:605–12.

13. Schrauzer, G. N. 1976. Selenium and cancer: A review. *Bioinorganic Chemistry* 5:275–81.

14. Chen, J., C. Geissler, et al. 1992. Antioxidant status and cancer mortality in China. *International Journal of Epidemiology* 21:624–35.

15. Potter, J. D., and K. Steinmetz. 1996. Vegetables, fruits and phytoestrogens as preventive agents. *Iarc Scientific Publications* 139:61–90.

16. Birt, D. F., and E. Bresnick. 1991. Chemoprevention by nonnutrient components of vegetables and fruit. In *Cancer and Nutrition*, R. B. Alfin-Slater and D. Kritchevsky, eds. New York: Plenum Press, 221–60.

17. Marwick, C. 1995. Learning how phytochemicals help fight disease. (Medical News & Perspectives) *Journal of the American Medical Association* 274:1328–30.

18. Dwyer, J. 1996. Is there a need to change the American diet? In *Dietary Phytochemicals in Cancer Prevention and Treatment*, American Institute for Cancer Research, ed. New York: Plenum Press, 189–98.

19. Brazelton, T. B., W. Dietz, and G. D. Comerci. 1995. Quoted in A. A. Skolnick, Experts debate food stamp revision. *Journal of the American Medical Association* 274:782.

Chapter 5 ~ The Wisdom of Herbs

1. Fransworth, N. R., and R. W. Morris. 1976. Higher plants—the sleeping giant of drug development. *American Journal of Pharmacy* 147:46–52.

2. Duke, J. A. 1997. Ethnobotany: The riches of medicinal plants. *Complementary Medicine for the Physician* 2:15.

3. Tyler, V. E. 1994. *Herbs of Choice.* New York: Pharmaceutical Products Press, 143–46.

4. Ames, B. N., R. Magaw, and L. S. Gold. 1987. Ranking possible carcinogenic hazards. *Science* 236:271–79.

5. Steinmuller, C., J. Roesler, et al. 1993. Polysaccharides isolated from plant cell cultures of Echinacea purpurea enhance the resistance of immunosuppressed mice against systemic infections with Candida albicans and Listeria monocytogenes. *International Journal of Immunopharmacology* 15:605–14.

6. Lau, B., H. C. Ruckle, et al. 1994. Chinese medicinal herbs inhibit growth of murine renal cell carcinoma. *Cancer Biotherapy* 9:153–61.

7. Budhiraja, R. D., and S. Sudhir. 1987. Review of biological activity of withanolides. *Journal of Scientific and Industrial Research* 40:488–91.

8. Mowrey, D. B., and D. E. Clayson. 1982. Motion sickness, ginger and psychophysics. *Lancet* 1 (March 20):655–57.

9. Schulz, H., C. Stolz, and J. Muller. 1994. The effect of valerian extract on sleep polygraphy in poor sleepers: A pilot study. *Pharmacopsychiatry* 27:147–51.

10. Arora, R. B., and B. R. Madan. 1965. Cardiovascular pharmacotherapeutics of six medicinal plants indigenous to India. *Award Monograph Series, Number 1*, Hamdard National Foundation, New Delhi, India.

11. Blass, E. M. and J. Blom. 1996. Beta-casomorphin causes hypoalgesia in 10–day-old rats: Evidence of central mediation. *Pediatric Research* 39:199–203.

Chapter 6 ~ Contending with Cancer

1. Singh, S. P., S. K. Abraham, and P. C. Kesavan. 1996. Radioprotection of mice following garlic pretreatment. *British Journal of Cancer* 74 (Supplement) 27:S102–S104.

2. Jin, R., L. L. Wan, and T. Mitsuishi. 1995. Effects of shi-ka-ron and Chinese herbs in mice treated with anti-tumor agent mitomycin C. *Chung Kuo Chung Hsi I Chieh Ho Tsa Chih* 15:101–3.

3. Chu, D. T., W. L. Wong, and G. M. Mavligit. 1988. Immunotherapy with Chinese medicinal herbs. II. Reversal of cyclophosphamide-induced immune suppression by administration of fractionated Astragalus membranceus in vivo. *Journal of Clinical and Laboratory Immunology* 25:125–29.

4. Khoo, K. S., and P. T. Ang. 1995. Extract of astragalus membranaceus and ligustrum lucidum does not prevent cyclophophamide-induced myelosuppression. *Singapore Medical Journal* 36:387–90.

5. Mitchell, M. S., W. Harel, et al. 1993. Active specific immunotherapy of melanoma with allogenic cell lysates. Rationale, result, and possible mechanisms of action. *Annals of the New York Academy of Science* 690:153–66.

6. Nicholson, S., C. S. R. Gooden, et al. 1998. Radioimmunotherapy after chemotherapy compared to chemotherapy alone in the treatment of advanced ovarian cancer: A matched analysis. *Oncology Reports* 5:223–26.

7. Vollmers, H. P., F. Hensel, et al. 1998. Tumor-specific apoptosis induced by the human monoclonal antibody SC-1: A new therapeutical approach for stomach cancer. *Oncology Reports* 5:35–40.

8. Jacobsen, P. B., D. H. Bovbjerg, et al. 1995. Conditioned emotional distress in women receiving chemotherapy for breast cancer. *Journal of Consulting and Clinical Psychology* 63:108–14.

9. Bovbjerg, D. H., and W. H. Redd. 1992. Anticipatory nausea and immune suppression in cancer patients receiving cycles of chemotherapy: Conditioned responses? In *Psychoneuroimmunology*, H. Schmoll, U. Tewes, N. P. Plotnikoff, eds. Lewiston, N.Y.: Hogrefe & Huber Publishers, 237–250.

10. Ader, R. 1975. Behaviorally conditioned immunosuppression. *Psychosomatic Medicine* 37:333–42.

11. Shibata, H., R. Fujiwara, et al. 1992. Restoration of immune function by olfactory stimulation with fragrance. *Psychoneuroimmunology*, H. Schmoll, U. Tewes, and N. P. Plotnikoff, eds. Lewiston, N.Y.: Hogrefe and Huber Publishers.

Chapter 7 ~ Envisioning Wholeness

1. Dossey, L. *Healing Words*. New York: HarperCollins.

2. French, A. P., J. Tupin, et al. 1981. Physiological changes with a simple relaxation method. *Psychosomatics* 22:794–801.

3. Wallace, R. K., and H. Benson. 1972. The physiology of mediation. *Scientific American* 226:84–90.

4. Massion, A. O., J. Teas, et al. 1995. Meditation, melatonin and breast/prostate cancer: Hypothesis and preliminary data. *Medical Hypothesis* 44:39–46.

5. Simonton, O. C., S. Matthews-Simonton, and J. Creighton. 1978. *Getting Well Again: A step-by-step, self-help guide to overcoming cancer for patients and their families.* Los Angeles: J. P. Tarcher.

Chapter 8 ~ Sensual Healing

1. Mehrabian, X., and X. Ferris. 1967. Inference in attitudes from nonverbal communication in two channels. *Journal of Consulting Psychology* 31:248–52.

2. Good, M. 1996. Effects of relaxation and music on postoperative pain: A review. *Journal of Advanced Nursing* 24:905–14.

3. Zimmerman, L., J. Nieveen, et al. 1996. The effects of music interventions on postoperative pain and sleep in coronary artery bypass graft (CABG) patients. *Scholarly Inquiry for Nursing Practice* 10:153–70.

4. Kaminski, J., and W. Hall. 1996. The effect of soothing music on neonatal behavioral states in the hospital newborn nursery. *Neonatal Network* 15:45–54.

5. Standley, J. M., and F. S. Moore. 1995. Therapeutic effects of music and mother's voice on premature infants. *Pediatric Nursing* 21:509–12.

6. Mornhinweg, C. G., and R. R. Voignier. 1995. Music for sleep disturbance in the elderly. *Journal for Holistic Nursing* 13:248–54.

7. Lowis, M. J., and J. Hughes. 1997. A comparison of the effects of sacred and secular music on elderly people. *Journal of Psychology* 131:45–55.

8. Belin, P., P. Van Eeckhout, et al. 1996. Recovery from nonfluent aphasia after melodic intonation therapy: A PET study. *Neurology* 47:1504–11.

9. Marwick, C. 1996. Leaving concert hall for clinic, therapists now test music's "charms." *Journal of the American Medical Association* 275:267–68.

10. Blumenstein, B., M. Bar-Eli, and G. Tenenbaum. 1995. The augmenting role of biofeedback: Effects of autogenic, imagery and music training on physiological indices and athletic performance. *Journal of Sports Sciences* 13:343–54.

11. Johnston, K., and J. Rohaly-Davis. 1996. An introduction to music therapy: Helping the oncology patient in the ICU. *Critical Care Nursing Quarterly* 18:54–60.

12. Keller, V. E. 1995. Management of nausea and vomiting in children. *Journal of Pediatric Nursing* 10:280–86.

13. Le Mée K. 1994. *Chant*. New York: Bell Tower.

14. Sabo, C. E., and S. R. Michael. 1996. The influence of personal massage with music on anxiety and side effects associated with chemotherapy. *Cancer Nursing* 19:283–89.

15. Field T. M., Schanberg S. M., et al. 1986. Tactile/kinesthetic stimulation effects on preterm neonates. *Pediatrics* 77:654–58.

16. Field, T. 1995. Massage therapy for infants and children. *Journal of Developmental and Behavioral Pediatrics* 16:105–11.

17. Scafidi, F., and T. Field. 1996. Massage therapy improves behavior in neonates born to HIV-positive mothers. *Journal of Pediatric Psychology* 21:889–97.

18. Field, T., N. Grizzle, et al. 1996. Massage and relaxation therapies' effects on depressed adolescent mothers. *Adolescence* 31:903–11.

19. Cady, S. H., and G. E. Jones. 1997. Massage therapy as a workplace intervention for reduction of stress. *Perceptual and Motor Skills* 84:157–58.

20. Dunn, C., J. Sleep, and D. Collett. 1995. Sensing an improvement: An experimental study to evaluate the use of aromatherapy, massage, and periods of rest in an intensive care unit. *Journal of Advanced Nursing* 21:34–40.

21. Curtis, M. 1994. The use of massage in restoring cardiac rhythm. *Nursing Times* 90:36–37.

22. Groer, M., J. Mozingo, et al. 1994. Measures of salivary secretory immunoglobulin A and state anxiety after a nursing back rub. *Applied Nursing Research* 7:2–6.

23. Ironson, G., T. Fields, et al. 1996. Massage therapy is associated with enhancement of the immune system's cytotoxic capacity. *International Journal of Neuroscience* 84:205–17.

24. Rhiner, M., B. R. Ferrell, et al. 1993. A structured nondrug intervention program for cancer pain. *Cancer Practice* 1:137–43.

25. Ferrell-Torry, A. T., and O. J. Glick. 1993. The use of therapeutic massage as a nursing intervention to modify anxiety and the perception of cancer pain. *Cancer Nursing* 16:93–101.

26. Jung, C. G. 1939. Dream symbols of the process of individuation. In *The Integration of the Personality*, C. G. Jung, ed. New York: Farrar & Rinehart, 96–204.

27. Argüelles, J., and M. Argüelles. 1972. *Mandala*. Berkeley, Calif.: Shambala, 53.

28. Redd, W., and S. Manne. 1991. Fragrance reduces patient anxiety during stressful medical procedures. *Focus on Fragrance*, Summer edition, 1.

29. Foreyt, J. P. 1970. Control of overeating by aversive therapy. *Dissertation Abstracts International* 30:5688.

30. Kumori, T., R. Fujiwara, et al. 1995. Effects of citrus fragrance on immune function and depressive states. *Neuroimmunomodulation* 2:174–80.

31. Buchbauer, G., L. Jirovetz, et al. 1993. Fragrance compounds and essential oils with sedative effects upon inhalation. *Journal of Pharmaceutical Sciences* 82:660–64.

32. Shibata, H., Fujiwara, R., et al. 1992. Restoration of immune function by olfactory stimulation with fragrance. In *Psychoneuroimmunology*, H. Schmoll, U. Tewes, and N. P. Plotnikoff, eds. Lewiston, N.Y.: Hogrefe & Huber Publishers, 161–171.

Healing Sounds Suggestions

Asher, J. 1995. *Feet in the Soil*. Boulder, Colo.: New Earth Records. (303) 444–9122.

BecVar, B., and B. BecVar. 1997. *The Magic of Healing Music*. San Rafael, Calif.: Shining Star Productions. (415) 456–6568.

The Benedictine Monks of Santo Domingo de Silos. 1982. *Chant*. Madrid, Spain: EMI Records.

Endangered Species. 1995. *Dancing in the Trance*. Sonoma, Calif.: Global Pacific Records.

Gordon, D. and S. 1996. *Sacred Spirit Drums*. Topanga, Calif.: Sequoia Records.

Gorn, S. 1994. *Luminous Ragas*. Brattleboro, Vt.: Interworld Music Associates.

Sachdev, G. S. 1995. *Vedic Music*. Sudbury, Mass. Infinite Possibilities. (800) 858–1808.

Chapter 9 ~ A Time to Every Purpose

1. Focan, C., D. Focan-Henrard, et al. 1986. Cancer associated alteration of circadian rhythms in carcinoembryonic antigen (CEA) and alpha-fetoprotein (AFP) in humans. *Anticancer Research* 6:1137–44.

2. Driessche, T. V. 1988. Research on the molecular basis of circadian rhythmicity. The cellular approach. In *Trends in Chronobiology*, W. T. J. M. Hekkens, G. A. Kerkhof, and W. J. Rietveld, eds. Oxford, Eng.: Pergamon Press, 19–29.

3. Irwin, M., A. Mascovich, et al. 1994. Partial sleep deprivation reduces natural killer cell activity in humans. *Psychosomatic Medicine* 56:493–98.

4. Lacoste, V., and L. Wetterberg. 1993. Individual variations of rhythms in morning and evening types with special emphasis on seasonal differences. In *Light and Biological Rhythms in Man*, L. Wetterberg, ed. Oxford, Eng.: Pergamon Press, 287–304.

5. Samel, A., H. M. Wegman, et al. 1991. Influence of melatonin treatment on human circadian rhythmicity before and after a simulated nine hour time shift. *Journal of Biological Rhythms* 6:235–48.

6. Society of light treatment and biological rhythms. 1990. Consensus statement on the efficacy of light treatment for SAD. *Light Treatment and Biological Rhythms Bulletin* 3:5–9.

7. Bartsch, H., C. Bartsch, et al. 1993. The relationship between the pineal gland and cancer: Seasonal aspects. In *Light and Biological Rhythms in Man*, L. Wetterberg, ed. Oxford, Eng.: Pergamon Press, 337–47.

8. Levi, F. 1994. Chronotherapy of cancer: Biological basis and clinical applications. *Pathologie Biologie* 42:338–41.

9. Focan, C. 1995. Circadian rhythms and cancer chemotherapy. *Pharmacology and Therapeutics* 67:1–52.

Chapter 10 ~ Emotional Healing

1. Grossarth-Maticek, R., and H. J. Eysenck. 1990. Personality, stress and disease: Description and validation of a new inventory. *Psychological Reports* 66:355–73.

2. Levenson, J. L., Bemis, C., and B. A. Presberg. 1994. The role of psychological factors in cancer onset and progression: A critical appraisal. In *The Psychoimmunology of Cancer*, C. E. Lewis, C. O'Sullivan and J. Barraclough, eds. New York: Oxford University Press, 246–64.

3. Baltrusch, H., W. Stangel, and M. Waltz. 1988. Cancer from the behavioral perspective: The type C pattern. *Activitaf Nervosa Superior* 30:18–20.

4. Pennebaker, J. W., J. K. Kiecolt-Glaser, and R. Glaser. 1988. Disclosures of traumas and immune function: Health implications for psychotherapy. *Journal of Consulting and Clinical Psychology* 56:239–45.

5. Petire, K. J., R. J. Booth, et al. 1995. Disclosure of trauma and immune response to a hepatitis B vaccination program. *Journal of Consulting and Clinical Psychology* 63:787–92.

6. Heim, E. Coping and adaptation in cancer. 1991. In *Cancer and Stress: Psychological, biological and coping studies*, C. L. Cooper and M. Watson, eds. Chichester, Eng.: John Wiley and Sons, 197–235.

7. Spiegel, D., J. Bloom, et al. 1989. Effect of psychosocial treatment on survival of patients with metastatic breast cancer. *Lancet* 2:888–91.

Chapter 11 ~ Healing through Expression

1. Jung, C. G. 1965. *Memories, Dreams, Reflections*. New York: Vintage Books, page 196.

2. Condon, W. S., and L. W. Sander. 1974. Neonate movement is synchronized with adult speech: Interactional participation and language acquisition. *Science* 183:99–101.

3. Pennebaker, J. W., J. K. Kiecolt-Glaser, and R. Glaser. 1988. Disclosures of traumas and immune function: Health implications for psychotherapy. *Journal of Consulting and Clinical Psychology* 56:239–45.

General References

Argüelles, J., and M. Argüelles. 1995. *Mandala*. Boston: Shambhala.

Chodorow, J. 1991. *Dance Therapy & Depth Psychology*. London: Routledge.

Feder, E., and B. Feder. 1981. *The Expressive Arts Therapies*. Englewood Cliffs, N.J.: Prentice-Hall, Inc.

Gilroy, A., and C. Lee. 1995. *Art and Music: Therapy and research*. London: Routledge.

Jung, C. G. 1964. *Man and His Symbols*. Garden City, N.J.: Doubleday.

Rogers, N. 1993. *The Creative Connection*. Palo Alto, Calif.: Science & Behavior Books, Inc.

Suggested Music for Movement Therapy Exercises

Classical

Bach, J. S. *Brandenburg Concertos 1–6*. Vienna Master Series. 1991. Munich, Ger.: Pilz Media Group.

Bach, J. S. *Concerto for Two Violins in D minor*. Yehudi Menuhin, violinist. 1995. London: Seraphim.

Beethoven, L. *Piano Sonata No. 8 "Pathétique."* Anton Dikov, pianist. 1990. Los Angeles: Delta Music.

Brahms, J. *Piano Concerto No. 1 in D minor, opus 15.* Second movement (Adagio). András Schiff, pianist. 1989. London: London Records.

Contemporary

Ciani, S. *Pianissimo.* 1990. Los Angeles: Private Music.

Franke, C. *Enchanting Nature.* 1994. West Hollywood, Calif.: Earthtone Records.

Halpern, S. *Gifts of the Angels.* 1994. San Anselmo, Calif.: Sound Rx.

Lanz, D. *Return to the Heart.* 1991. Milwaukee, Wis.: Narada Productions.

Chapter 12 ~ The Best Medicine

1. Ames, L. B. 1949. Development of interpersonal smiling response in the pre-school years. *Journal of Genetic Psychology* 74:273–91.

2. Kenderdine, M. 1931. Laughter in the pre-school child. *Child Development* 2:228–30.

3. Maclean, I. 1994. Dr. Rabelais's 500 year old prescription. *British Medical Journal* 308:803–4.

4. Cousins, N. 1976. Anatomy of an Illness as Perceived by the Patient. *New England Journal of Medicine* 295:1458–63.

5. Cousins, N. 1979. *Anatomy of an Illness as Perceived by the Patient.* New York: W. W. Norton.

6. Berk, L., S. Tan, et al. 1989. Neuroendocrine and stress hormone changes during mirthful laughter. *American Journal of the Medical Sciences* 298:390–96.

7. Berk, L. 1996. The laughter-immune connection: New discoveries. *Humor and Health Journal* 5:1–5.

8. Yoshino, S., J. Fuhimori, and M. Kohda. 1996. Effects of mirthful laughter on neuroendocrine and immune systems in patients with rheumatoid arthritis. *Journal of Rheumatology* 23:793–94.

9. Spiegel, K. P. 1972. Early conceptions of humor. In *The Psychology of Humor,* J. H. Goldstein and P. E. McGhee, eds. New York: Academic Press, 4–34.

10. Gelkopf, M., S. Kreitler, and M. Sigal. 1993. Laughter in a psychiatric ward. Somatic, emotional, social and clinical influences on schizophrenic patients. *Journal of Nervous and Mental Disease* 181:283–89.

11. Weisenberg, M., I. Tepper, and J. Schwarzwald. 1995. Humor as a cognitive technique for increasing pain tolerance. *Pain* 63:207–12.

12. Osho. 1992. *Meditation—The First and Last Freedom.* Cologne, Ger.: Rebel Publishing House, 47–50.

13. Robbin, T. 1984. *Jitterbug Perfume.* New York: Bantam Books, 380–81.

Chapter 13 ~ Weighing the Options

1. Eisenberg, D. M., R. C. Kessler, et al. 1993. Unconventional medicine in the United States: Prevalence, costs and patterns of use. *New England Journal of Medicine* 328:246–52.

2. Elder, N. C., A. Gillcrist, and R. Minz. 1997. Use of alternative health care by family practice patients. *Archives of Family Medicine* 6:181–84.

3. Cassileth, B. R. 1986. Unorthodox cancer medicine. *Cancer Investigation* 4:591–98.

4. Bailar, J. C. and H. L. Gornik. 1997. Cancer undefeated. *New England Journal of Medicine* 336:1569–74.

5. Mowrey, D. B., and D. E. Clayson. 1982. Motion sickness, ginger and psychophysics. *Lancet* 1 (March 20):655–57.

6. Field, T. M., S. M. Schanberg, et al. 1986. Tactile/kinesthetic stimulation effects on preterm neonates. *Pediatrics* 77:654–58.

7. Green, S. 1992. A critique of the rationale for cancer treatment with coffee enemas and diet. *Journal of the American Medical Association* 268:3224–27.

8. Rowinsky, E. K. 1997. The development and clinical utility of the taxane class of antimicrotubule chemotherapy agents. *Annual Review of Medicine* 48:353–74.

9. Moertel, C. G., T. R. Fleming, et al. 1982. A clinical trial of amygdalan (Laetrile) in the treatment of human cancer. *New England Journal of Medicine* 306:201–6.

10. Mathews, J. 1992. Sharks still intrigue cancer researchers. *Journal of the National Cancer Institute* 84:1000–1002.

11. O'Regan, B., and C. Hirshberg. 1993. *Spontaneous Remission: An annotated bibliography.* Sausalito, Calif.: Institute of Noetic Sciences

12. Cherkin, D. C., and F. A. MacCornack. 1989. Patient evaluation of low back pain care from family physicians and chiropractors. *Western Journal of Medicine* 150:351–55.

13. Koes, B. W., L. M. Bouter, et al. 1992. A blinded randomized clinical trial on manual therapy and physiotherapy for chronic back and neck complaints: Physical therapy measures. *Journal of Manipulative and Physiological Therapeutics* 15:16–23.

14. Coan, R. M., G. Wong, and P. L. Coan. 1980. The acupuncture treatment of low back pain: A randomized controlled study. *American Journal of Chinese Medicine* 9:326–32.

15. Christensen, P. A., M. Noreng, et al. 1989. Electroacupuncture and postoperative pain. *British Journal of Anaesthesia* 62:258–62.

16. Vincent, C. A. 1989. A controlled trial of the treatment of migraine by acupuncture. *Clinical Journal of Pain* 5:305–12.

17. Dundee, J. W., J. Yang, and C. McMillan. 1991. Non-invasive stimulation of the P-6 (Neiguan) antiemetic acupuncture point in cancer chemotherapy. *Journal of the Royal Society of Medicine* 84:210–12.

18. Fisher, P., A. Greenwood, et al. 1989. Effects of homeopathic treatment on fibrositis (fibromyalgia). *British Medical Journal* 299:365–66.

19. Reilly, D. T., C. McSharry, et al. 1986. Is homeopathy a placebo response? Controlled trial of homeopathic potencies, with pollen in hayfever as a model. *Lancet* 2:881–86.

20. Gipson, R. G., S. L. M. Gipson, et al. 1980. Homeopathic therapy in rheumatoid arthritis: Evaluation by double-blind clinical therapeutic trial. *British Journal of Clinical Pharmacology* 9:453–59.

21. Davenas, E., F. Beauvais, et al. 1988. Human basophil degranulation triggered by very dilute antiserum against IgE. *Nature* 333:816–18.

General References

Diamond, W. J., W. L. Cowden, with B. Goldberg. 1997. *An Alternative Medicine Definitive Guide to Cancer.* Tiburon, Calif.: Future Medicine Publishing. (An extensive survey of alternative approaches to cancer with a strong antiestablishment, pro-alternative perspective.)

Fugh-Berman, A. 1996. *Alternative Medicine: What Works.* Tucson, Ariz.: Odonian Press. (A very readable and balanced survey of published scientific research on alternative medicine.)

Jacobs, J., ed. 1996. *The Encyclopedia of Alternative Medicine.* Boston: Journey Editions. (A user-friendly guide to alternative approaches with beautiful photographs.)

Chapter 14 ~ Holistically Specific

1. Parker, S. L., T. Tong, et al. 1977. Cancer statistics, 1997. *CA—A Cancer Journal for Clinicians* 47:5–27.

2. Ziegler, R. G., R. N. Hoover, et al. 1993. Migration patterns and breast cancer risk in Asian-American women. *Journal of the National Cancer Institute* 85:1819–27.

3. Cohen, L. A., D. O. Thompson, et al. 1986. Dietary fat and mammary cancer II. Modulation of serum and tumor lipid composition and tumor prostaglandins by different dietary fat: Association with tumor incidence patterns. *Journal of the National Cancer Institute* 77:43–51.

4. Prentice, R., D. Thompson, et al. 1990. Dietary fat reduction and plasma estradiol concentration in healthy postmenopausal women. *Journal of the National Cancer Institute* 82:129–34.

5. Peterson, G., and S. Barnes. 1996. Genistein inhibits both estrogen and growth factor-stimulated proliferation of human breast cancer cells. *Cell Growth and Differentiation* 7:1345–51.

6. Lockwood, K., S. Moesgaard, and K. Folkers. 1994. Partial and complete regression of breast cancer in patients in relation to dosage of coenzyme Q10. *Biochemistry and Biophysics Research Communication* 199:1504–08.

7. Lockwood, K., S. Moesgaard, et al. 1995. Progress on therapy of breast cancer with vitamin Q10 and the regression of metastases. *Biochemistry and Biophysics Research Communication* 212:172–77

8. Pienta, K. J., and P. S. Esper. 1993. Risk factors for prostate cancer. *Annals of Internal Medicine* 118:793–803.

9. Hill, P., E. L. Wynder, et al. 1979. Diet and urinary steroids in black and white North American men and black South African men. *Cancer Research* 39:5101–5.

10. Morton, M. S., A. Matos-Ferreira, et al. 1997. Measurement and metabolism of isoflavonoids and lignans in the human male. *Cancer Letters* 114:145–51.

11. Stephens, F. O. 1997. Phytoestrogens and prostate cancer: Possible preventive role. *Medical Journal of Australia* 167:138–40.

12. Gann, P. H., C. H. Hennekens, et al. 1994. Prospective study of plasma fatty acids and risk of prostate cancer. *Journal of the National Cancer Institute* 86:281–86.

13. Giovannucci, E., A. Ascherio, et al. 1995. Intake of carotenoids and retinol in relation to risk of prostate cancer. *Journal of the National Cancer Institute* 87:1767–76.

14. Clinton, S. K., C. Emenhiser, et al. 1996. Cis-trans lycopene isomers, carotenoids, and retinol in the human prostate. *Cancer Epidemiology and Biomarks Preview* 5:8223–33.

15. Muir, C., J. Waterhouse, et al. 1987. Cancer incidence in five continents. *International Agency for Research on Cancer (IARC) Volume 5 (No. 88)*. Lyon, France.

16. Maziere, S., P. Cassand, et al. 1997. Vitamin A and apoptosis in colonic tumor cells. *International Journal for Vitamin and Nutrition Research* 67:237–41.

17. Reddy, B. S., A. Rivenson, et al. 1997. Chemoprevention of colon cancer by organoselenium compounds and impact of high- or low-fat diets. *Journal of the National Cancer Institute* 89:506–12.

18. Lipkin, M., H. L. Newmark, and G. Kelloff, eds. 1991. *Calcium, Vitamin D and Prevention of Colon Cancer*. Boca Raton, Fla.: CRC Press.

19. Sikorski, R., and R. Peters. 1997. Oncology ASAP—Where to find reliable cancer information on the Internet. *Journal of the American Medical Association* 277:1431–32.

Chapter 15 ~ The Unknown Destination

1. Kübler-Ross, E. 1969. *On Death and Dying*. New York: Macmillan Publishing Company.

2. Stern, C., Liturgy Committee of the Central Conference of American Rabbis. 1979. *Gates of Repentance*. New York: Central Conference of American Rabbis and Union of Liberal and Progressive Synagogues, 251.

3. Phillips, D. P., and E. W. King. 1988. Death takes a holiday: Mortality surrounding major social occasions. *Lancet* 2:728–32.

4. Phillips, D. P., and D. G. Smith. 1990. Postponement of death until symbolically meaningful occasions. *Journal of the American Medical Association* 263:1947–51.

5. Easwaran, E. 1987. Death as teacher: The Katha Upanishad. *The Upanishads.* Tomales, Calif.: Nilgiri Press, 86.

6. Moody, R. A. 1975. *Life after Life.* New York: Bantam Books.

7. Ring, K. 1980. *Life at Death.* New York: Coward, McCann and Geoghegan.

8. Sabom, M. B., and S. Kreutziger. 1977. The experience of near death. *Death Education* 1:195–203.

9. Ring, K. 1982. Frequency and stages of the prototypic near-death experience. In *A Collection of Near-Death Research Reading*, C. R. Lundahl, compiler. Chicago: Nelson-Hall Publishers, 110–47.

10. Moody, R. A. 1982. The experience of dying. In *A Collection of Near-Death Research Reading*, C. R. Lundahl, compiler. Chicago: Nelson-Hall Publishers, 89–109.

11. Drab, K. J. 1981. The tunnel experience: Reality or hallucination? *Anabiosis* 1:126–52.

12. Greyson, B. 1993. Varieties of near-death experience. *Psychiatry* 56:390–99.

13. Owens, J. E., E. W. Cook, and I. Stevenson. 1990. Features of "near-death experience" in relation to whether or not patients were near death. *Lancet* 336:1175–77.

14. Kellehear, A. 1996. Near-death experiences across cultures. In *Experiences Near Death.* New York: Oxford University Press, 22–41.

15. Thurman, R. A. F., trans. 1994. *The Tibetan Book of the Dead.* New York: Bantam Books.

16. Tagore, R. *Wings of Death—The Last Poems of Rabindranath Tagore.* Translated from the Bengali by Aurobindo Bose. London: Butler & Tanner LTD. (Note: This poem was sung at Tagore's commemoration service after his death for the first time.)

General References

Barton, D. 1977. *Dying and Death—A clinical guide for caregivers.* Baltimore: Williams & Wilkins Company.

Basford, T. K. 1990. *Near-Death Experiences—An annotated bibliography.* New York: Garland Publishing.

Kalish, R. A. 1958. *Death, Grief, and Caring Relationships.* Monterey, Calif.: Brooks/Cole Publishing Company.

Kastenbaum, R. J. 1991. *Death, Society, and Human Experience.* New York: Macmillan Publishing Company.

Kübler-Ross, E. 1975. *Death—The final stage of growth.* Englewood Cliffs, N.J.: Prentice-Hall.

Lundahl, C. R., compiler. 1982. *Collection of Near-Death Research Reading.* Chicago: Nelson-Hall Publishers.

Nuland, S. B. 1995. *How We Die.* New York: Vintage Books.

Postscript

1. Bailar, J. C., and H. L. Gornik. 1997. Cancer undefeated. *New England Journal of Medicine* 336:1569–74.

2. Wingo, P. A., L. A. Ries, et al. 1998. Cancer incidence and mortality, 1973–1995. A report card for the U.S. *Cancer* 82:1197–1207.

Index